The Effective Health Care Program of the Agency for Healthcare Research and Quality (AHRQ) conducts and supports research focused on the outcomes, effectiveness, comparative clinical effectiveness, and appropriateness of pharmaceuticals, devices, and health care services. More information on the Effective Health Care Program can be found at www.effectivehealthcare.ahrq.gov.

This report was produced under contract to AHRQ by the University of North Carolina at Chapel Hill under Contract No. 290-2010-000141. The AHRQ Task Order Officer for this project was Parivash Nourjah, Ph.D. The findings and conclusions in this document are those of the authors, who are responsible for its contents; the findings and conclusions do not necessarily represent the views of AHRQ. Therefore, no statement in this report should be construed as an official position of AHRQ or of the U.S. Department of Health and Human Services.

This report may be used, in whole or in part, as the basis for development of clinical practice guidelines and other quality enhancement tools, or as a basis for reimbursement and coverage policies. AHRQ or U.S. Department of Health and Human Services endorsement of such derivative products may not be stated or implied.

This document is in the public domain and may be used and reprinted without permission except those copyrighted materials that are clearly noted in the document. Further reproduction of those copyrighted materials is prohibited without the specific permission of copyright holders.

Persons using assistive technology may not be able to fully access information in this report. For assistance contact EffectiveHealthCare@ahrq.hhs.gov.

> None of the investigators have any affiliations or financial involvement that conflicts with the material presented in this report.

Suggested citation: Dusetzina SB, Tyree S, Meyer AM, Meyer A, Green L, Carpenter WR. Linking Data for Health Services Research: A Framework and Instructional Guide. (Prepared by the University of North Carolina at Chapel Hill under Contract No. 290-2010-000141.) AHRQ Publication No. 14-EHC033-EF. Rockville, MD: Agency for Healthcare Research and Quality; September 2014. www.effectivehealthcare.ahrq.gov/reports/final.cfm.

Linking Data for Health Services Research: A Framework and Instructional Guide

Prepared for:

Agency for Healthcare Research and Quality
U.S. Department of Health and Human Services
540 Gaither Road
Rockville, MD 20850
www.ahrq.gov

Contract No. 290-2010-000141

Prepared by:

The University of North Carolina at Chapel Hill
Chapel Hill, NC

Authors:

Stacie B. Dusetzina, Ph.D.
Seth Tyree, M.S., M.A.
Anne-Marie Meyer, Ph.D.
Adrian Meyer, M.S.
Laura Green, M.B.A.
William R. Carpenter, Ph.D.

AHRQ Publication No. 14-EHC033-EF
September 2014

Acknowledgments

This project was funded by the Agency for Healthcare Research and Quality under contract number 290-2010-000141 (Developing and Evaluating Methods for Record Linkage and Reducing Bias in Patient Registries). The authors would like to acknowledge the University of North Carolina Lineberger Comprehensive Cancer Center and the University Cancer Research Fund for facilitating the data acquisition. They would also like to thank the Technical Expert Panel Members, and the ICISS staff and faculty collaborators, without whom this report would not be possible (http://iciss.unc.edu/team.php).

Contents

Chapter 1. Background and Purpose 1
    Overview 1
    Background 1
    Purpose 2

Chapter 2. Research Environment 5
    Overview 5
    Computing Systems and the Balance Between Security and Usability 5
        Desktop Computer: High Security, Low Usability, Low Cost 6
        Central Server: Medium Security, Medium Usability, Moderate Cost 6
        Virtual Remote Desktops: High Security, High Usability, High Cost 6
    Building the Technical Platform 6
        Securing the Platform 7
        Users Accessing Platform 7
        Gaining Access to Platform 7
        Processing Power of Platform 7
        Data Storage Platform 7
    Securing the Research Environment 8
        Overview 8
        Regulatory Requirements 8
        Identifying Sensitive Data 9
        Summary of Protected Information 11
        Building and Implementing a Security Plan 12
        Workforce Training 12
    Managing Risks 13
        Identifying and Assessing Risk 13
        Tracking Risks 14
        Planning Risk Responses 14
        Implementing Risk Responses 16
        Monitoring Risks 16
    Conclusions 16
    Appendix 2.1. Procedures and Processes To Enhance Data Security 17

Chapter 3. Linkage Feasibility--To Link or Not To Link 21
    Overview 21
    Evaluating Linkage Feasibility 21
    Purpose and Conditions for Original Data Collection 23
    Ownership of Data 24
    Data Sharing and Security Concerns 25
    Methods for Privacy Protection in Record Linkage 26
    Building the Team 27

Chapter 4. An Overview of Record Linkage Methods 29
    Overview 29
    Data Cleaning and Standardization 29
    Linkage Methods 31
        Deterministic Linkage Methods 32
        Probabilistic Linkage Methods 33
    Alternative Linkage Methods 36
    Selecting a Linkage Method 36
    Evaluating Linkage Algorithms 36
    Validating Linkage Results 37
    Final Remarks 38
    Appendix 4.1. Useful SAS Functions and Procedures 41
    Appendix 4.2. Data Linkage Software Packages 49

Chapter 5. Evaluation of Methods Linking Health Registry Data to Insurance Claims in Scenarios of Varying Available Information 51
    Objective 51
    Methods 51
        Approach Overview 51
        Data Sources and Patient Populations 52
        Data Cleaning and Standardization 53
        Data Linkage 53
    Results 56
        Gold-Standard Linkage 56
        Deterministic Linkage 57
        Probabilistic Linkage 59
    Discussion 62
    Appendix 5.1. SEER-Medicare Algorithm With Partial Identifiers 63

Chapter 6. Project Summary and Recommendations for Researchers 65
Overview 65
Considerations for Project Planning 65
    Appropriateness and Feasibility of the Project 65
    Data Ownership and Governance 65
    Technical Environment and Security 66
    Team, Skills, and Expertise 66
    Cost 66
    Identification and Evaluation of Available Linkage Keys 66
    Variable Cleaning, Standardization, and a Common Data Model (Normalization) 67
    Linkage Approach 67
    Evaluation and Validation of Record Linkage 68
    Recommendations for Reporting Results 68
    Framework for Registry-to-Claims Linkage 69
    Project Planning Checklist 69
    Project Execution Checklist 69

References 71

Abbreviations 77

Figures
Figure 2.1. Security versus usability 5
Figure 2.2. Component architecture 6
Figure 2.3. Risk-management cycle 13
Figure 2.4. Process for creating a merged dataset 18
Figure 2.5. Physical storage areas 19

Tables
Table 2.1. Example of matrix summarizing protected information types 11
Table 2.2. Example of risk scores 14
Table 2.3. Example of generic risk register 15
Table 3.1. Linkage identifiers 21
Table 4.1. Common variations found in selected linkage identifiers 30
Table 4.2. True match status by algorithm output 36
Table 5.1. Overview of experimental linkage approach 52
Table 5.2. Variables available for linkage and their completeness in study datasets 52
Table 5.3. Example md5 algorithm values from inconsistent strings 55
Table 5.4. Selected results of gold-standard linkage algorithm with partial identifiers 56
Table 5.5. Selected results of deterministic linkage algorithms 58
Table 5.6. Selected results of deterministic linkage algorithms using encrypted data 60
Table 5.7. Selected results of probabilistic linkage algorithms 61

Chapter 1. Background and Purpose

Overview

Health registries greatly enhance health services research, especially when linked with other data sources such as administrative claims. Recently, concerns about patient privacy and data security have produced policies such as the Health Insurance Portability and Accountability Act (HIPAA) that reduce the availability of sensitive identifying information. In this context, the development of effective record linkage approaches for varying scenarios of data availability is critical. This report presents a conceptual framework and instructional information that scientifically describe the strengths and limitations of different approaches to record linkage of registries to other data sources. This chapter presents the context and motivation for the work detailed in subsequent chapters. Specifically, it describes the need for data linkages in general, and linkages of registries to health insurance claims specifically, in the context of comparative effectiveness research (CER) and the environments in which CER is conducted.

Background

Randomized controlled trials (RCTs) remain the gold standard for assessing intervention efficacy; however, RCTs are not always feasible or sufficiently timely. Perhaps more importantly, RCT results often cannot be generalized due to a lack of inclusion of "real-world" combinations of interventions and heterogeneous patients.[1-4] With recent advances in information technology, data, and statistical methods, there is tremendous promise in leveraging ever-growing repositories of secondary data to support comparative effectiveness and public health research.[2,5-6] Observational studies of secondary data can help fill the knowledge gaps unaddressed by RCTs and extend the utility of current data investments by examining important research questions and health care programs. Because of this, the Institute of Medicine and others have strongly advocated for CER using secondary data from sources such as health registries, administrative claims, and electronic health records.[7-10]

Although these secondary data sources have many strengths, they also have important limitations. For example, because they are often collected for nonresearch purposes, secondary datasets do not have the benefit of randomization to control for confounders (factors associated with treatment and outcomes) that threaten to bias study findings.[11-13] Moreover, individual datasets are often limited in scope, which in turn limits their utility in addressing important questions in a comprehensive manner. Some limitations can be overcome by linking data from multiple sources.[7,14-16] Linking a registry with external data can facilitate case and control group identification, improve measurement of risk factors and outcomes, and allow passive followup of study participants.[13,17-19] Linkages can also be used to refine and validate measures created using claims data or other registries[20-22] or to adjust for unmeasured confounding by using supplemental data about a subset of observations.[23] However, data linkage from multiple sources in support of CER and public health research continues to face several challenges.

Data linkage involves pairing observations from two or more files and identifying the pairs that belong to the same entity.[24] A common form of linkage is to collect information on the same person from two datasets. However, linkage errors can arise from multiple points when data sources are inconsistent in capturing the same person, a person's records do not link due to missing or inaccurate data in one or more files, or different people are erroneously linked for the same reasons.[12] The causes of these errors are many, including poor data quality, data sources that use different systems for coding the linking variables in their records, inadequate capacity of linking software to handle large datasets, and complexity of data linking systems that have substantial learning curves. These factors can be compounded by recent policy changes that restrict access to key linking variables.

For public health and health care delivery settings, concerns regarding privacy, confidentiality, and safety have led to increasingly stringent policies and regulations governing the collection, use, and transfer of Personally Identifiable Information. Perhaps the most well-known patient privacy policy is HIPAA, which has been widely decried by health care programs and researchers as exemplifying the law of unintended consequences. Intended to protect patients from misuse of their personal information, the law has been associated with a substantially greater burden for both health care providers and researchers, and even indicted as contributory to patient deaths and research bias that may misinform and thus diminish the quality of future health care delivery.[25-30] Indeed, a recent consensus report by the Institute of Medicine contends that HIPAA, passed with the intention of protecting patient privacy, does not protect privacy as well as it should, and agrees with assertions that HIPAA impedes important research.[31] Policies such as HIPAA have severely limited access to unique identifiers (e.g., Social Security Numbers, names), traditional mainstays of quality data linkages involving person-level data,[32-34] and many programs have even stopped collecting some identifying information.

In addition to concerns about availability of unique identifiers across datasets, there are several notable concerns regarding the datasets themselves. The validity threats due to nonrandomization include confounding by indication (treatment assignment influenced by risk for the outcome), selection bias (due to inability to define an appropriate control group), and misclassification of exposures or outcomes. Additionally, linkage errors can systematically bias effect estimates.[11-13] Although researchers have continued to develop new methods for deterministic and probabilistic linkage, alternative methods have not been tested thoroughly and comprehensive guidelines are lacking.[11,35-36]

In light of these challenges, there is an urgent need to develop greater knowledge of how to perform reliable valid linkages to support the integration of disease registry and administrative data for health services research. Such linkages are important for leveraging the investment already made on the collection of the individual data sources and allowing their use for examining important CER and public health questions. Without such gains in knowledge and capacity, health care programs will miss substantial opportunities to use vastly expanding data resources to improve the public's health, and many stakeholders will remain skeptical of clinical or policy decisions based on incomplete data.[37-39]

Purpose

This report serves as a conceptual framework for data linkage in the context of CER. The report defines the requirements for high-quality record linkage of registries to other data sources and describes the strengths and limitations of different approaches. By explaining the spectrum of activities involved, it serves as an instructional guide for researchers designing new CER studies using patient registries linked with other secondary data sources. Through this report, we provide an overview of linkage from registries to administrative claims, including considerations for researchers, data managers, information technology managers, and other stakeholders who are likely to be involved in the process of data linkage. We also apply the data linkage framework to a real-world problem and discuss the results.

This report is informed by practical insight developed by researchers affiliated with the AHRQ (Agency for Healthcare Research and Quality) DEcIDE (Developing Evidence to Inform Decisions about Effectiveness) CER Consortium, who acquire, maintain, and link sensitive secondary data to support CER and outcomes research studies. Consistent with the goals of AHRQ and the DEcIDE Network, this report will enhance the ability of CER/patient-

Chapter 1. Background and Purpose

centered outcomes research to inform consumers, clinicians, policymakers, and other health care decisionmakers.

Record linkage in support of CER is more than simply joining two datasets. Rather, it is an extensive process that involves many steps and collaborations among multiple partners. Researchers hoping to link data sources should first be aware of the technical, legal, and data-management challenges and considerations. The remaining chapters in this report are designed to prepare researchers by providing them with the information necessary for high-quality data linkage.

Chapter 2 describes the components of a secure research environment. It is set in the context of building trust among data/research partners and includes technical and administrative guides to establishing a secure computing platform enabling sophisticated CER research. Additionally it discusses approaches to secure confidentiality, integrity, and availability of data in order to maintain compliance with State and Federal regulations.

Chapter 3 describes general considerations that must be addressed when planning to link data. The focus spans issues pertaining to requesting, receiving, and managing data from different sources; Data Use Agreements/Contracts; data ownership; and deciding whether data linkage is feasible and appropriate.

Chapter 4 guides the reader through an overview of data linkage methods in an effort to document a set of best practices for conducting linkages and recommendations for evaluating and reporting the validity and reliability of the linkage procedure selected. It begins with issues pertaining to the quality of the available linkage keys—specifically, completeness, overlapping information, and commonly observed idiosyncrasies. It focuses on the creation of a common data model via techniques for cleaning and standardizing the linkage keys before linkage. Next, an overview of data linkage methods is provided, including a detailed summary of deterministic and probabilistic linkage methods as well as techniques for evaluating the quality of the linkage. Finally, this chapter includes a set of appendixes that contain (1) lists and characteristics of several open-source and commercial software packages for data linkage, (2) sample SAS code for data preparation and linkage, and (3) recommended readings for those interested in learning more about alternative methods.

Chapter 5 presents an approach to linking registry data to administrative claims using the methods discussed in Chapter 4. Our approach involves four components: (1) employment of a gold standard, (2a) evaluation of deterministic approaches, (2b) evaluation of a deterministic approach using encryption, and (3) probabilistic approaches, each applied in varying scenarios of data availability to ascertain optimal approaches in given scenarios. In step 2b, a deterministic approach using encryption, we simulate a scenario of restrictions on identifier release to researchers. Given the exceptionally limited availability of practical empirical examples researchers can use to inform their own data linkages, this chapter articulates specific examples in depth, detailing the steps researchers may take and what they may expect to find given their unique scenarios of data availability and data quality.

Finally, Chapter 6 summarizes the report and provides specific recommendations for researchers who plan to undertake a data linkage project. We also provide information, including a checklist, for researchers to use in both the project planning phase and the project execution phase.

Chapter 2. Research Environment

Overview

A foundational element of any research project is the research program environment. In the context of comparative effectiveness research (CER) using linked data, a secure and well-performing environment is important for several reasons, including that it helps build and assure trust between researchers and the providers of sensitive data, be they patients, registry administrators, insurance claim administrators, or others. If data providers are confident that a research partner has strong administrative and technical security systems and takes data security seriously at a programmatic level, they will be more confident in providing sensitive data to the researchers, including data with unique identifiers. As we describe in Chapters 4 and 5 of this report, linkage quality is typically much stronger when unique identifiers are available. Therefore, a secure research environment and capable information technology support can directly influence the quality of the research data obtained and, by extension, research results. With faith in the integrity and security of the research environment, data providers may also be more likely to provide other unique data that can be important to driving truly innovative research.

A secure and well-performing environment is also important in that system performance and security controls can directly influence the scope of the research project, including the size and complexity of the data that can be managed and linked to support the project. Often, as the scope and complexity of research projects increase and the data volume grows, computing environments are challenged to scale up to ensure seamless operations.

This chapter describes key considerations concerning the research environment, including the technical platform and security considerations, to guide researchers as they seek to develop or optimize their systems for CER projects using large volumes of data such as linked registry and administrative claims data.

Computing Systems and the Balance Between Security and Usability

As shown in Figure 2.1, security and usability often stand on opposite ends of a spectrum. The tradeoff for having a highly secure system is decreased accessibility and practical usability, whereas systems that are highly accessible often face greater challenges in assuring data security. Understanding the scope of the research project and the needs of the researcher or research team is important to specifying a system configuration that meets the needs of the project and balances security with usability. For example, a single researcher with a small research project of limited scope will likely have different needs for a computing environment compared with a large decentralized research team undertaking a multiyear research study using national data.

Figure 2.1. Security versus usability

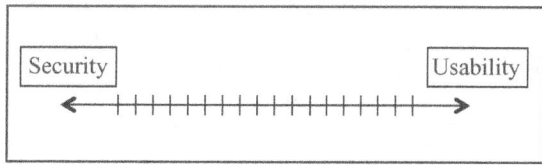

We present three different computing system scenarios to help researchers identify where on the spectrum their program may fall. While this discussion does not take into account the number of users, it is important to note that the cost of large systems varies greatly depending on existing infrastructures and purchasing prices of solutions offered by various vendors.

Desktop Computer: High Security, Low Usability, Low Cost

In this environment, the user accesses all data on a dedicated desktop computer located in a dedicated and constantly locked office with limited network access.

- *Security*: The risks of theft and network attacks are reduced to a minimum.
- *Usability*: Multiple users will never be able to access the data concurrently.

Central Server: Medium Security, Medium Usability, Moderate Cost

This environment allows multiple users to connect remotely through a secure command line (e.g., through a secure protocol such as SSH) to a central computing server housing all the data and tools.

- *Security*: The risk increases while gaining access to information over a network. Controlling individual users' access to information creates new administrative challenges.
- *Usability*: Multiple users can collaborate on a central system. Computing jobs can be submitted in the background and the progress can be checked from remote locations.

Virtual Remote Desktops: High Security, High Usability, High Cost

This environment allows multiple users to connect remotely to virtualized desktops over the Internet from laptops or desktop computers to access shared data and tools.

- *Security*: Since the accessing computers supply only monitor, keyboard, and mouse, the data never leave the server environment. Even secure printing to dedicated printers is possible to control paper output.
- *Usability*: Each user connects to a virtual computer in the central environment. All tools are housed on the server but accessed through existing desktops.

Building the Technical Platform

Regardless of the selected technologies, the number of users, or security requirements, the technical platform can be disassembled into various components (Figure 2.2). Defining the requirements for the individual components creates a meaningful information technology plan.

Figure 2.2. Component architecture

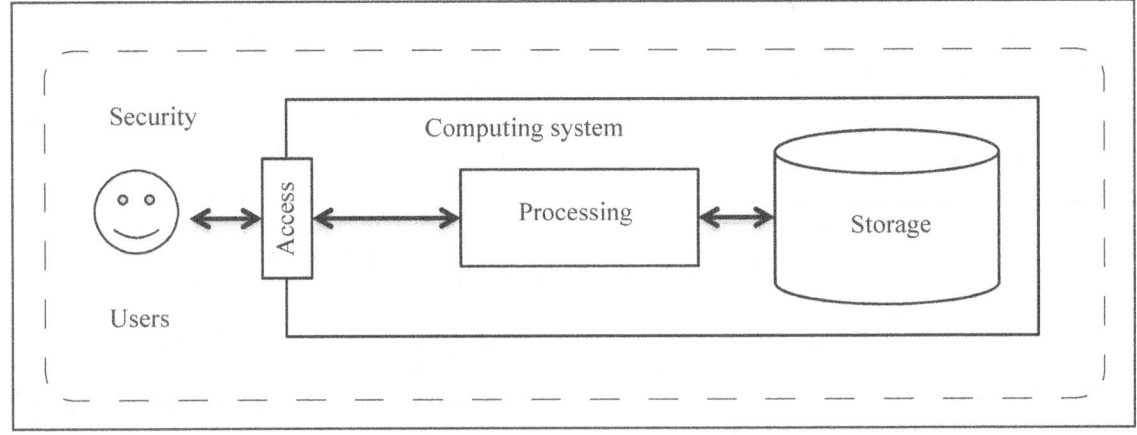

Chapter 2. Research Environment

Securing the Platform

Most regulatory security frameworks, such as the Health Information Portability and Accountability Act (HIPAA) and Federal Information Security Management Act (FISMA), focus on controlling the confidentiality, integrity, and availability of information. The efforts to implement administrative, physical, and technical safeguards tend to scale up as the system complexity increases. Regulatory requirements and risk assessments will strongly affect the technical implementations.

Users Accessing Platform

To support a wide range of innovative research on complex linked data resources, the experience and focus of team members narrow and deepen. Work is divided among individuals to cover areas such as data management, data linking, cohort discovery, advanced modeling, and more. Complex research projects depend on the seamless integration and collaboration of the various users and the use of their preferred tools. By defining the user profiles and job responsibilities, the main usability properties of the expected environment are established. Examples of typical roles within complex project teams include the following.

Role: Data Manager. The data manager takes care of the data. This might include importing new data, conversion of file formats, preparation and receipt of data carriers (storage devices), archiving obsolete data, and granting access to data.

Role: Data Linking. The linking expert is responsible for linking data sources. This might include cleaning linking variables, building linking methods, and cohort discovery (e.g., selection of patients meeting specific study-inclusion criteria), resulting in datasets for various research projects.

Role: Analyst/Statistician. The statistician is responsible for all modeling aspects of a research study. These might include creating analytic cohorts for study questions (using previously linked deidentified data), preparing data for modeling, and analyzing data to meet project objectives.

Gaining Access to Platform

Access management controls how users gain access to the system and data. An existing organization might have a central user-management process that establishes authentication with a simple username/password combination. More advanced two-factor authentication methods ensure that a compromised password alone does not convey access to the system. Biometric authentication (e.g., fingerprint reader) verifies the identity of the intended user. Examples of commonly used authentication methods and their pros and cons are provided in Appendix 2.1.

Processing Power of Platform

The processing power of the computing system directly affects the time it takes to manipulate the data. As linking processes touch the same information repeatedly, tuning parameters to optimize the performance of hardware and software will reduce the run times. For considerations for hardware performance, see Appendix 2.1.

It is important to understand that the researcher's network has an impact on data flow. The network can quickly become the bottleneck for moving data, resulting in an exceptionally slow response. In an optimized setup, the connection between data and processing components is a dedicated Gigabit (1,000Mbps) network or even fiber optics. Any components between the processing and storage, such as firewalls, network switches, or routers, will reduce information flow. In a setup in which the data are stored on hard drives directly attached to the processing system, network performance will have a limited impact on data flow.

Data Storage Platform

The storage performance directly affects the time it takes to perform data tasks. For example, tasks such as cleaning and standardizing data, combining data sources, or performing exploratory analyses of linked data sources are storage-intensive activities. The main technical characteristics of the storage platform are size and speed. A storage device is attached using a specific technology, such as Serial Advance Technology Attachment (SATA), Serial Attached Small Computer System Interface (Serial SCSI or SAS), Universal Serial Bus (USB), or Storage Area Network (SAN). Various vendors sell enterprise storage solutions encapsulating multiple storage devices in a single appliance.

Storage Size. When purchasing data carriers, it is important to understand that physical data size and actual available data size will greatly vary depending on the installation. Methods used to prevent data loss, such as Redundant Array of Independent Disks (RAID), might require as much as twice the amount of physical space as required for storing the physical data. The file system used to store data also affects available data size. A data carrier is divided into blocks like a blank book with many pages. The size of the data block is fixed for the entire file system. As an example, if the block size is 1,024 characters (or bytes) and a file of 1,500 characters is saved, it will consume 2,048 physical bytes on the data carrier. Since the partially used blocks cannot be used for other files, these bytes are "lost."

Storage Speed. Storage devices have two speed-related properties: (1) the time it takes to find the data on the carrier (referred to as seek time and measured in milliseconds) and (2) the continuous read/write performance. The seek time depends mainly on how fast the disk is spinning. Common rotation speeds are 5,400, 7,200, 10,000, and 15,000 revolutions per minute (RPM). In the case of a solid state disk (SSD), the seek time will be extremely low, as there are no moving parts. The continuous read/write performance depends not only on how fast the disk is spinning, but also on how the disk is attached to the processing system.

A well-performing storage system can read/write information at rates of 100MB/s or more. A disk spinning at 5,400 or 7,200 RPM, as delivered in standard laptops or desktops, generally cannot achieve this. In comparison, an SSD attached over SATA can easily reach read/write rates of 500MB/s or more. To optimize cost, a computing system can be outfitted with slower/cheaper storage for archiving in combination with fast analytic storage to support powerful processing.

Securing the Research Environment

Overview

Federal and State laws have mandated several sets of regulations, each intended to address one or more of the following objectives:

- **Confidentiality**: Preserving authorized restrictions on information access and disclosure, including means for protecting personal privacy and proprietary information
- **Integrity**: Guarding against improper information modification or destruction; includes ensuring information nonrepudiation and authenticity
- **Availability**: Ensuring reliable and timely access to information

Regulatory Requirements

The research environment must comply with applicable laws to protect the hosted information. Because HIPAA governs health information collected by covered entities mainly during health encounters, alternative research datasets might require compliance with other contractual requirements or State regulations. Researchers should consult with a regulatory expert as early as possible to ensure that they understand the scope of all applicable laws.

Regulatory requirements generally describe *what* must be controlled and leave it up to the research team to define *how* to reach the required controls by implementing adequate policies and procedures. Some State-level privacy laws may govern even self-collected information. In the following sections, we describe a sample of regulatory requirements that might be applicable to researchers working with sensitive health information.

Federal Information Security Management Act of 2002. FISMA defines a mandatory framework for managing information security for all information systems used or operated by a U.S. Federal Government agency or by a contractor or other organization on behalf of a Federal agency. It requires the development, documentation, and implementation of an information security program. The National Institute for Standards and Technology (NIST) standards and guidelines (Special Publications 800 series) and Federal Information Processing Standards (FIPS) publications further define the framework of the program.

Health Information Portability and Accountability Act. The U.S. Congress created HIPAA in 1996. Security standards establishing requirements to safeguard Protected Health Information (PHI), both paper and electronic (ePHI), were issued as part of HIPAA in April 2003. The security requirements specifically address administrative, physical, and technical safeguards meant to ensure that patient health records and Personally Identifiable Information (PII) remain as secure as possible.

State Security-Breach Laws. Forty-six States, the District of Columbia, and multiple U.S. territories (Guam, Puerto Rico, and the Virgin Islands) have enacted privacy-breach notification laws. While these laws can vary from State to State, they generally follow a similar framework. This framework defines "sensitive data," sets out requirements for triggering the breach-notification process, identifies actors and roles in the notification process, defines to whom the law applies, and describes those cases under which certain parties and/or information may be exempt from notification requirements (www.fas.org/sgp/crs/misc/R42475.pdf). Researchers are responsible for understanding their responsibilities under the relevant State breach-notification legislation and should consult legislative resources such as the National Conference of State Legislatures for regulatory text (www.ncsl.org).

Identifying Sensitive Data

Sensitive data are the information protected by regulatory requirements. The definition of sensitive data varies widely between laws. In some cases, the scope of a Data Use Agreement (DUA) could even require aggregation or define minimum cell sizes. In the following section, we provide a summary of regulatory definitions per FISMA, HIPAA, and State security-breach laws.

Personally Identifiable Information, FISMA. As used in information security, PII is any information maintained by an agency that can be linked to an individual. This includes (1) any information (e.g., name, Social Security Number, date and place of birth, mother's maiden name, or biometric records) that can be used to distinguish or trace an individual's identity and (2) any other information (e.g., medical, educational, financial, and employment information) that is linked or linkable to an individual. Examples of PII include, but are not limited to—

- Name, such as full name, maiden name, mother's maiden name, or alias

- Personal identification number, such as Social Security Number, passport number, driver's license number, taxpayer identification number, or financial account or credit card number

- Address information, such as street address or email address

- Personal characteristics, including photographic image (especially of face or other identifying characteristic), fingerprints, handwriting, or other biometric data (e.g., retina scan, voice signature, facial geometry)

Protected Health Information, HIPAA. The HIPAA Privacy Rule protects all "individually identifiable health information" held or transmitted by a covered entity or its business associate in any form or media, whether electronic, paper, or oral.

The Privacy Rule calls this information *Protected Health Information*, or PHI.

Under HIPAA, *individually identifiable health information* is information, including demographic data, that relates to any of the following:

- The individual's past, present, or future physical or mental health condition
- The provision of health care to the individual
- The past, present, or future payment for the provision of health care to the individual
- Information that identifies the individual or for which there is a reasonable basis to believe it can be used to identify the individual

Individually identifiable health information includes many common identifiers (e.g., name, address, birth date, Social Security Number). The Privacy Rule excludes from PHI employment records that a covered entity maintains in its capacity as an employer, and educational and certain other records subject to or defined in the Family Educational Rights and Privacy Act, 20 U.S.C. §1232g.

Electronic Protected Health Information, HIPAA. The HIPAA Security Rule protects a subset of information covered by the Privacy Rule, which is all individually identifiable health information a covered entity creates, receives, maintains, or transmits in electronic form. The Security Rule calls this information electronic *Protected Health Information*, or ePHI. The Security Rule does not apply to PHI transmitted orally or in writing.

Limited Datasets, HIPAA. HIPAA also has a provision for Limited Datasets (LDSs) from which most but not all potentially identifying information has been removed. Elements in an LDS are often necessary for research; however, *Direct Identifiers*, a subset of PHI defined by HIPAA §164.514(e)(2), must be removed. The Direct Identifiers include—

- Name
- Postal address information other than town or city, State, and ZIP Code
- Telephone numbers
- Fax numbers
- Electronic mail addresses
- Social Security Numbers
- Medical record numbers
- Health plan beneficiary numbers
- Account numbers
- Certificate/license numbers
- Vehicle identifiers and serial numbers, including license plate numbers
- Device identifiers and serial numbers
- Web Universal Resource Locators (URLs)
- Internet Protocol (IP) addresses
- Biometric identifiers, including finger and voice prints
- Full-face photographic images and any comparable images

LDSs can include the following PHI:

- Date of birth
- Date of death
- Dates of service
- Town or city
- State
- ZIP Code

Personal Information, State Security-Breach Laws. Researchers should review applicable State legislation for definitions of Personal Information. Generally, these definitions do not vary substantially from State to State and are very similar to Federal definitions. For example, the North Carolina State Security-Breach Laws (North Carolina General Statute §75-65) define Personal Information as a person's first name or first initial and last name in combination with any of the following identifying information:

- Social Security Number or employer taxpayer identification numbers

- Driver's license, State identification card, or passport numbers
- Checking account numbers
- Savings account numbers
- Credit card numbers
- Debit card numbers
- Personal Identification Number (PIN)
- Electronic identification numbers, electronic mail names or addresses, Internet account numbers, or Internet identification names
- Digital signatures
- Any other numbers or information that can be used to access a person's financial resources
- Biometric data
- Fingerprints
- Passwords
- Parent's legal surname before marriage

Summary of Protected Information

The research team may find it useful to summarize in matrix form the protected information types identified by applicable regulatory requirements. This matrix will help the research team identify information in datasets and assess the policies and procedures that might apply to a specific work task. Table 2.1 shows an example of one such matrix.

Table 2.1. Example of matrix summarizing protected information types

Identifying Information	Sensitive Data Type	
	Personal Information	Direct Identifiers
Name (full name/maiden name/mother's maiden name/alias)	X	X
Address information		X
Telephone/fax information		X
Personal IDs (SSN/taxpayer ID/driver's license number/State ID/passport number/birth date/certification or license numbers)	X	X
Financial IDs (checking/savings account numbers/PINs/credit card numbers)	X	X
Electronic IDs (email name/address/Internet account numbers/Internet ID/passwords)	X	X
Personal characteristics (digital signatures/biometric data/fingerprints/handwriting/full-face images)	X	X
Health care data/provisions/payment/beneficiary information (past, present, or future)		X
Employment information		X
Device IDs/serial numbers		X
Vehicle IDs		X

PIN = Personal Identification Number; SSN = Social Security Number.

Building and Implementing a Security Plan

Meeting applicable regulatory requirements requires thoughtful planning and management. While it is tempting to think of information security in terms of technological controls, successful security management requires people, processes, and technology in equal proportion. An overarching security management plan addresses how people, processes, and technology will be leveraged to maintain the confidentiality, integrity, and availability of sensitive data within the bounds set by applicable regulatory requirements.

While development of the security management plan is an iterative process, with sections added or refined as planning activities proceed, the document will ultimately address the following:

- *Security laws and regulations* describe those regulatory requirements applicable to the research team, as discussed previously.
- *Major functions* list those functions the security plan is intended to accomplish.
- *Scope* lists those sensitive data types the security program is intended to address.
- *Roles and responsibilities* describe roles that will be held by members of the organization and their responsibilities vis-à-vis information security.
- *Management commitment* represents an official statement on the part of the applicable management body in support of the processes and procedures documented within the security plan.
- *FISMA security categorization and impact level* define the FISMA category assigned to the data and information systems covered by the security plan. This section is applicable only to those systems subject to FISMA.
- *Compliance and entity coordination* describe which roles are responsible for ensuring organizational compliance with the security plan and which roles are responsible for coordinating security activities among relevant entities external to the research team (e.g., data centers, overarching security offices).
- *Implementation and governing plans* describe, at a high level, the number and content of all security subplans, defining the processes and procedures for—
  - Security documentation control
  - Risk management (described in further detail below)
  - Workforce security
  - Access management
  - Security training
  - Incident reporting
  - Contingency planning
  - Security assessment
  - Facility access
  - Workstation access
  - Devices and removable media
  - Data integrity
  - Authentication
  - Network security
  - System activity review/audit

At the outset of security planning, the research team should be able to define the security laws and regulations, major functions, and scope sections. Roles and responsibilities, management commitment, entity coordination, and FISMA categorization (if applicable) can be defined further through stakeholder meetings. The processes and procedures documented in the subplans will be developed as part of the risk-management process described below.

Workforce Training

A training plan defines working procedures, emergency and incident management, sanction policies, policies and procedures on how to inform members of the workforce about their roles and responsibilities, and other relevant procedures. Many large research environments might be able to leverage existing training modules. These might include training on HIPAA, research ethics, basic computer and network use, and basic human resources policies. Keeping the retraining on an annual basis is advisable.

Managing Risks

Research teams must first understand regulatory requirements, then select and implement adequate security controls to meet these requirements and to mitigate risks posed to the security of the organization's information systems and data. Often, discussions of information security mistakenly emphasize specific technical safeguards. An emphasis on risk management, however, properly defines technical solutions as the means by which organizational risks are controlled. Risk management, therefore, drives information security planning. A comprehensive risk-management program not only allows data custodians to identify risks posed to their data, but also provides a framework for selection of functional and technical security controls.

Data custodians subject to FISMA requirements should consult NIST guidance for implementing a FISMA-compliant life-cycle program, which includes detailed volumes of guidance and controls. We illustrate a more general risk-management framework in Figure 2.3. This framework envisions risk management as a continuous cycle of assessing, addressing, and monitoring organizational risk to ensure the confidentiality, integrity, and availability of information systems.

Identifying and Assessing Risk

Risk identification is conducted on any technology, process, and procedure within the scope of the environment. Risk identification is, simply put, the process of identifying and documenting potential threats to the research team's information and information systems. Risk identification can be conducted in a variety of ways, including brainstorming sessions, documentation reviews, assumptions analysis, cause and effect diagramming, strengths/weaknesses/opportunities/threats (SWOT) analysis, and expert consultation. Inclusion of an independent third party, be it an outside consultant or even representatives from a separate group within the research team, will provide an external point of view invaluable in fully defining the spectrum of potential adverse events. Regardless of the method used, this process must clearly identify and document the source of the risk and the impact of the risk should it be realized.

Figure 2.3. Risk-management cycle

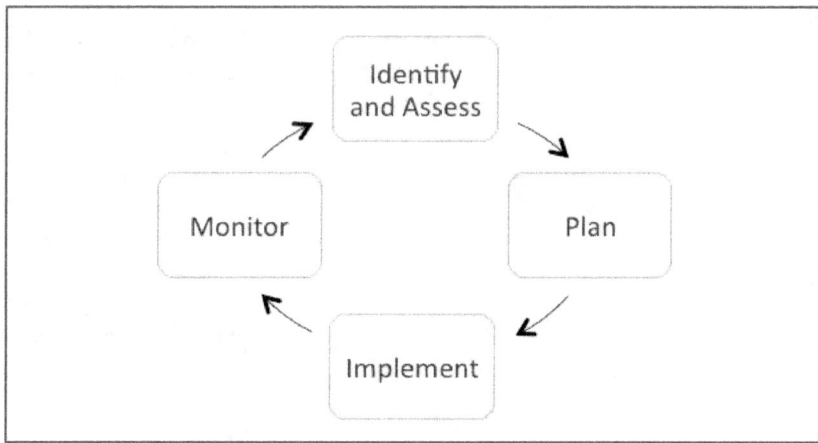

Assess identified risks along two primary dimensions: probability of occurrence and criticality of impact. Actions and mitigations planned in the next phase of the risk-management cycle will be based largely on each risk's score as assessed during this phase.

Risk scores evaluate the combination of the probability and impact of a security breach/incident. Higher scores represent higher security risks. Lower scores represent reduced security risks. Table 2.2 provides an example of how to plot and assess the severity of a security breach/incident (criticality of impact) and the likelihood of occurrence of an event.

Table 2.2. Example of risk scores

		Criticality of Impact		
		Low	Medium	High
Probability of Occurrence	High	3	6	9
	Medium	2	4	6
	Low	1	2	3

Examples of impact:

Loss of data
Loss of public confidence
Potential lawsuit
Multiplier effect

Examples of occurrence:

Frequency of information access
Number of users
Size of dataset

Tracking Risks

The risk register is the collection of all identified risks, their assessed impact and probability, and possible actions/mitigations. Both HIPAA and FISMA mandate the analysis of risk and a record thereof. Table 2.3 is an example of a generic risk register.

Planning Risk Responses

Once risks have been identified, assessed, and documented in the risk register, data custodians and other stakeholders can plan appropriate methods of dealing with each risk. Risk responses can be divided into four categories: avoidance, acceptance, transfer, and mitigation.

- *Risk avoidance* occurs when a research team takes the necessary actions to reduce the likelihood of risk realization to close to (if not exactly) zero. Generally, risk avoidance is the most desirable method of dealing with risks; however, it is often cost prohibitive or simply infeasible to avoid all risks.

- *Risk acceptance* occurs when a research team chooses to accept the consequences of a risk should it be realized. Risk acceptance is generally recommended when the impact of a risk is small or when the probability of occurrence is significantly lower than the cost to avoid, transfer, or mitigate. Each research team must define its own criteria for what constitutes an "acceptable" risk.

- *Risk transfer* occurs when a research team passes the impact of risk realization on to another party. The most common form of risk transfer is insurance. Risk transfer is feasible only when the impact can be clearly measured and addressed by the third party.

- *Risk mitigation* occurs when a research team takes steps to reduce the probability or impact of risk realization. Risks that cannot be avoided, accepted, or transferred must be mitigated.

After a research team decides whether to avoid, accept, transfer, or mitigate a risk, it must determine the necessary steps to do so. At this juncture, the research team will identify the necessary and appropriate technical controls to either avoid or mitigate certain risks. Actions identified in this phase must also be documented in the risk register.

Table 2.3. Example of generic risk register

Risk ID#	Score	Title	Description	Impact	Impact Score	Probability Score	Action
R001	6	Equipment stolen from office site	An individual gains access to office and removes electronic equipment.	Leak of data; through loss of computers, access to secure systems might be compromised.	High	Med	Lock building, encrypt data, alarm system
R002	3	Network access	An individual gains access to the network within the organization.	Leak of data; stolen passwords; computers connected to network are subject to hack or sniff attacks.	High	Low	Network firewalls, internal switched network, virus software, secure wireless
R003	6	Remote support	Support staff member gains access to an organizational computer for remote support purposes.	Leak of data; open connections to protected systems and open windows displaying PHI are visible to support individual.	Med	High	Configure to no auto desktop sharing; close applications with PHI
R004	6	Computer crash or upgrade	A computer used to access PHI stops working or is upgraded.	Leak of data; leak of passwords; old hard drive might get reused; warranty traded or sold.	High	Med	Disk encryption; disposition policy; no saving of passwords; use password management software
R005	2	Lack of DUA understanding	DUA limitations might be misinterpreted.	Violation of contract; misuse of data; leak of data.	Low	Med	Governance; DUA clarification and training
R006	2	Unauthorized staff gains access to data	Staff, students, collaborators, reviewers gain access to data protected by DUA.	Violation of contract; misuse of data; leak of data.	Low	Med	Administrative safeguards, training
R007	6	Data emailed for review	Protected data are shared through email; electronic documents within the intent of review.	Leak of data; violation of contract; information is no longer housed in secure environments.	Med	High	Secure email; training in email use; secure drop box
R008	2	Data emailed to incorrect individual	An email with protected information is sent to an unintended recipient.	Leak of data.	Low	Med	Email training; secure drop box

DUA = Data Use Agreement; Med = medium; PHI = Protected Health Information.

Implementing Risk Responses

During the implementation phase, the research team develops and deploys the technical controls identified in the planning phase. Just as importantly, the research team must also document the controls selected, develop all necessary records, and train stakeholders accordingly. Users must understand not only how to use any security controls implemented but also the "rules of behavior" for maintaining a secure environment. Technical controls alone are not sufficient to create a fully secure environment; users and other stakeholders must foster and maintain a *culture* of security.

Monitoring Risks

Risk management is an ongoing cyclical process. The research team must periodically reassess the environment for new or changing risks, which in turn must be identified, assessed, and addressed through planning and action. Thoughtful and frequent monitoring of risk allows a research team to adapt more easily to changes, both expected and unexpected, without compromising information security.

Conclusions

A research environment incorporating a secure and well-performing computing platform represents the operational backbone for conducting innovative research using complex linked data sources. Securing and safeguarding the information not only meets legal and regulatory requirements, but also builds needed trust among stakeholders. Data providers will be more open to providing access to their information, researchers will be confident in accessing sensitive data, and programmers and analysts will operate effectively in a standardized environment with consistent application of technologies and tools. The technical implementation, combining performance and storage, will enable complex data management, as described in Chapter 3. Supported by the leadership, successfully implemented security policies and procedures fit seamlessly into daily workflows, reducing and mitigating potential risks. The environment is now ready to support research and to receive even the most sensitive data.

Appendix 2.1. Procedures and Processes To Enhance Data Security

Moving Sensitive Data Using CDs or DVDs

Perform the following steps to create and transport sensitive data using CDs or DVDs. This procedure can be adapted for electronic transfer using a protocol such as the secure file transfer protocol (SFTP).

1. Create a new media number and add it to a data carrier list tracking all movable media containing sensitive data.
2. Create a local folder with the media number as the name.
3. Assemble all the data in the created folder.
4. Generate an encryption key using a GUID (globally unique identifier) tool such as that found at www.guidgenerator.com/ and print it on a document along with the media number.
5. Create an archive using a PGP (http://en.wikipedia.org/wiki/Pretty_Good_Privacy) encryption tool with all the contents of the folder, using the GUID as the encryption key.
6. After testing the self-extracting archive, use a file-shredding tool (www.fileshredder.org/) to remove the folder with the data.
7. Burn the archive onto a data CD or DVD labeled with the media number.
8. You can now mail the data carrier, and fax or email the encryption key separately to the receiving party.

Guidelines for Storage and Destruction of Movable Media

- Store movable media in a safe, separated from the encryption keys.
- Destroy damaged and/or retired media, including hard disks, by shredding.
- Update movable media records for every media item that is disposed of or destroyed.
- Shred any printed material at location or use a secure document disposal service.

Decoupling and Mapping Data

Figure 2.4 describes a process for adding data sources to the research data environment, removing direct identifiers, and creating a merged dataset with elements regarding the individuals' health status or health services utilization. In the context described below, we retain Protected Health Information (PHI) within the original data files but limit access (a process known as decoupling). When PHI is destroyed following the data linkage, this is known as deidentification. We use the terms *deidentified* and *decoupled* interchangeably in this report as we discuss data security and staging, but readers should understand the differences represented by the terminology.

Figure 2.4. Process for creating a merged dataset

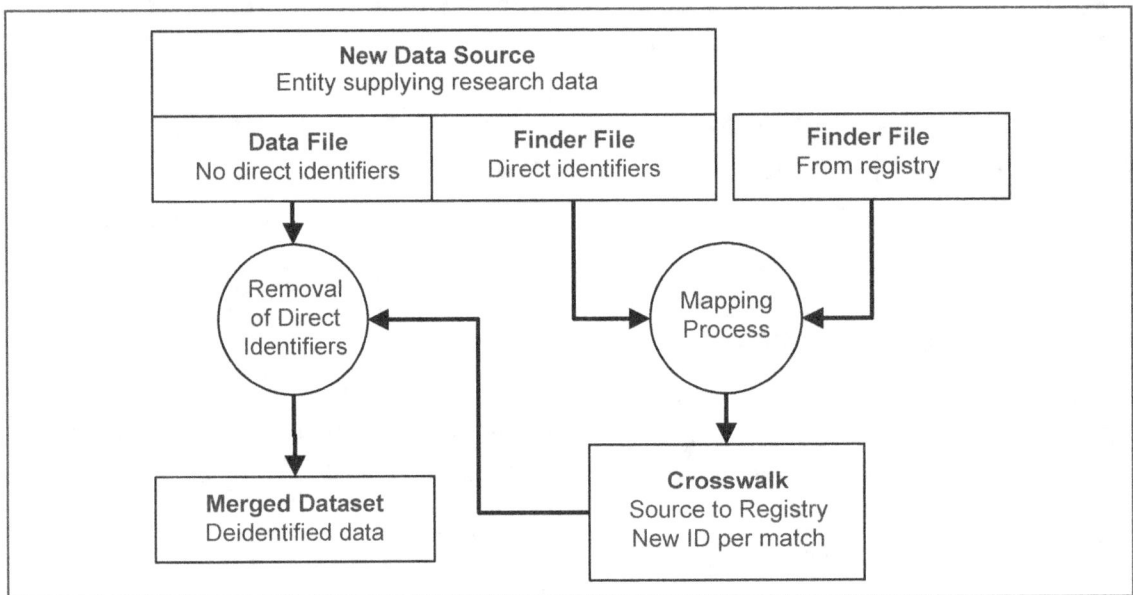

Data file: This file contains raw data such as claims, diagnoses, and treatment. Individuals cannot be directly identified in these data.

Finder file: The finder files contain direct identifiers of individuals.

Mapping process: Using a mapping method, the individuals in the finder files are matched.

Crosswalk: The crosswalk identifies matching records for each individual and possible duplicates. A new unique identifier (ID) is assigned for each true identified research subject.

Removal of direct identifiers: Using the crosswalk and the data file, a new file is generated by replacing the source identifiers with the new IDs.

Merged dataset: Information about an individual can now be accessed across data sources and deidentified datasets using the new IDs.

Physical Separation of Data Using Storage Architecture

In the computing environment, data are separated physically into the three storage areas, as shown in Figure 2.5.

Appendix 2.1. Procedures and Processes To Enhance Data Security

Figure 2.5. Physical storage areas

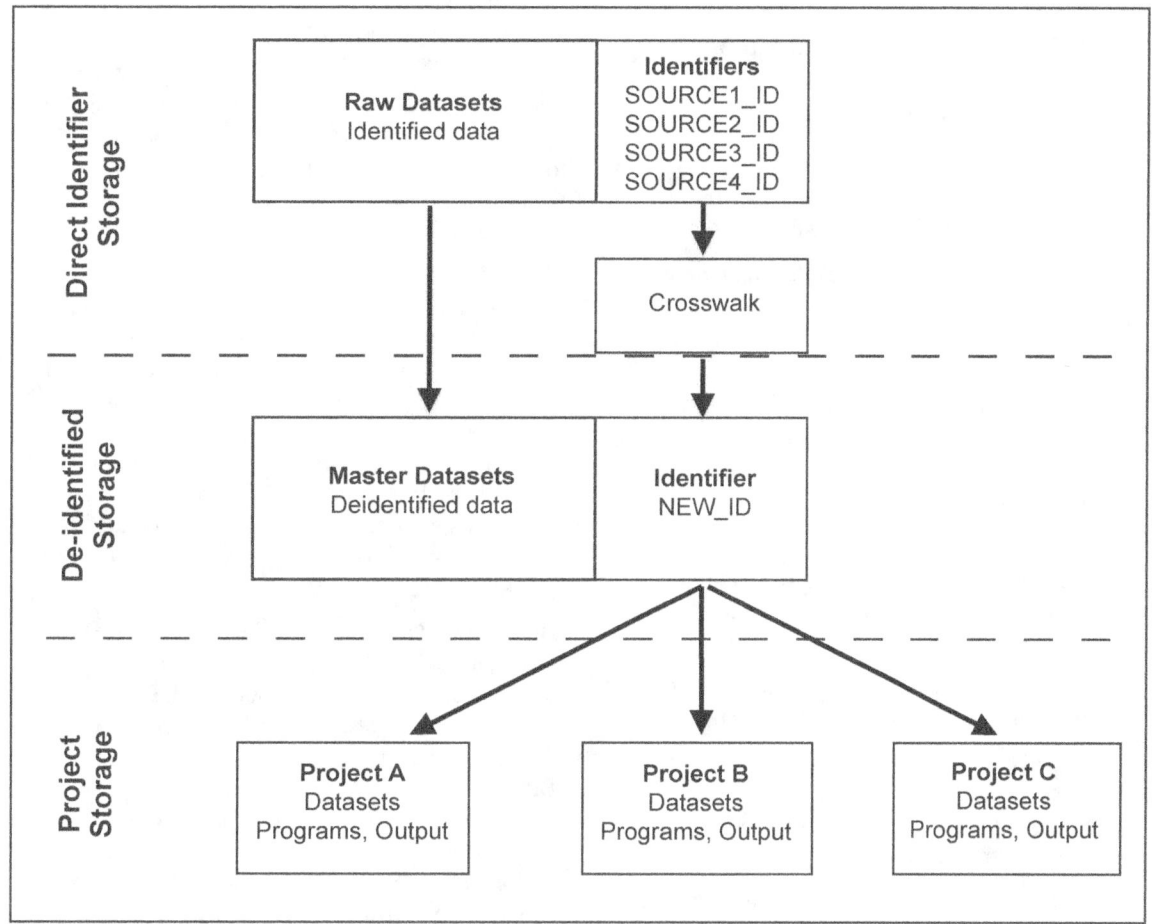

Direct identifier storage: Raw data including direct identifiers are secured in a highly restricted part of the system. The *direct identifier* space is accessible only through very restrictive access-management controls. All work on data linking and removal of direct identifiers is performed in this environment. Only a limited set of specifically trained, authorized individuals work in this environment.

Deidentified storage: The *deidentified* space contains deidentified master datasets from each source. This storage might be accessible to authorized users in read-only mode. Research datasets are extracted, or "cut," from these master files.

Project storage: Individual programmers access this space for projects. Institutional Review Boards and Data Use Agreements control the access to master datasets and datasets for projects.

Examples of Common Authentication Methods

Simple User Account. A user authenticates with username and password.

- *Pros*: This is a quick and simple way to access a system.
- *Cons*: Once the username and password are known, any individual can gain access.

Two-Factor Authentication. A user authenticates with username, password, and Personal Identification Number (PIN) (e.g., RSA secure ID).

- *Pros*: A changing PIN provides a second factor in addition to logging in with the username and password. An authentication is not possible without the device.
- *Cons*: The PIN verification is costly and, depending on the implementation, requires that the computing environment have access to the system verifying the PIN.

Biometric Authentication. A user authenticates with username, password, and (for example) a fingerprint.

- *Pros*: The additional biometric verification requires the account holder to be present at the time of authentication.
- *Cons*: Managing biometric information requires custom software installations on the client system.

Performance Considerations for Computer Hardware

Fine-tuning the three hardware components of memory, central processing unit (CPU), and bus speed is essential for the actual processing power. Random access memory (RAM) can be added after a purchase, but changes to the CPU or bus speeds are complicated and impractical. The bus speed represents how fast information can be moved between the CPU and the memory, and from and to the attached storage. When purchasing a system, you should purchase the highest affordable CPU/bus speed combination while leaving space to add memory later.

Central Processing Unit. Performance of a CPU is affected by (a) sockets (i.e., actual number of CPUs); (b) cores and threads (i.e., how instructions can be processed in parallel); and (c) clock (i.e., a number in GHz representing how many instructions are processed per second).

Random Access Memory. Selecting memory is dependent on the supported architecture of the motherboard. Manufacturers generally advise on what type of memory is supported and best for optimized performance. The product description of memory often includes physical and performance parameters. For example "240-Pin DDR3 1600" represents memory that has 240 pins connecting it to the motherboard and supports a 1600MHz clock.

Bus Speed. Depending on the architecture, there are multiple bus speeds affecting data throughput between storage, memory, and CPU. For example: a hard disk might be attached using SATA3 or "SATA 6Gb/s," representing a bus speed of 6Gb/s. Bus speeds on the CPU/motherboard (chipset layout) are more complicated and fine-tuned by the vendor. Components with fancy names such as North Bridge, South Bridge, and Front Side Bus (FSB) (http://en.wikipedia.org/wiki/Front-side_bus) are part of this architecture. Vendors typically offer systems with high-performance options where these speeds are optimized and enhanced compared with home use products.

Chapter 3. Linkage Feasibility—To Link or Not To Link

Overview

In this chapter, we provide an overview of factors that researchers should consider before embarking on a data linkage project. These include:

1. Determining the feasibility of data linkage through assessing variable overlap and data quality
2. Determining the original purpose of the data and whether the terms of the original data collection prohibit the linkage
3. Determining data ownership, regulatory requirements, and limitations on use
4. Planning for data sharing and managing data security concerns
5. Ensuring that a qualified team is available to manage data security and the technical aspects of the data linkage

Because of the importance of each of these steps, researchers ideally should evaluate these concerns to the extent possible before applying for grant funding. (See Chapter 6 for a checklist with preliminary planning steps.)

Evaluating Linkage Feasibility

A fundamental step in any linkage effort is the prospective assessment of linkage feasibility. The feasibility of a linkage project depends largely on the quantity and quality of the identifying information available in the data sources being linked.[40]

Identifiers, full or partial, are more or less informative depending on their discriminatory power, or number of unique values. For instance, month of birth, which has 12 unique values, is more informative than sex, which has only 2 unique values. Assuming uniform distributions, record pairs matched randomly will agree on sex 50 percent (1/2) of the time simply by chance, while record pairs matched randomly will agree on month of birth 8.3 percent (1/12) of the time. Thus, when a matched pair agrees on month of birth, it is less likely that the pair matched simply by chance and more likely that the pair matched because the records represent the same individual. In this sense, month of birth contains more information than sex. Combining identifiers further increases the number of unique values (or "pockets"), thereby decreasing the chances that two records will match by chance alone. Table 3.1 shows identifiers commonly used for record linkage.

Table 3.1. Linkage identifiers

Type of Identifier	Variable Description
Unique patient identifiers	Social Security Number Medical record number Patient/beneficiary identification number
Indirect identifiers	Name: first, last, middle, maiden, alias Dates: birth, death, diagnosis, treatment, admission, discharge Sex Geographic location: street, city, county, ZIP, State Diagnosis codes

Additional information can be gleaned from the values themselves—that is, matches on rarely occurring values are less likely to occur by chance than matches on frequently occurring values. For instance, a match on a rarely occurring surname such as Lebowski is less likely to occur by chance than a match on a frequently occurring surname such as Smith. Because of this, a match on a rarely occurring surname, compared with a match on a frequently occurring surname, increases confidence that a matched pair is a true match.

Before embarking on a linkage project, it is important to consider whether a reliable and accurate linkage is possible given the available identifiers and their discriminatory power. Potential data quality issues that cannot be known before receiving the data prevent us from knowing this for certain. For instance, every beneficiary in an administrative health plan claims database may have a Social Security Number (SSN) captured, but we cannot know ahead of time whether the SSN was entered correctly or whether it represents the given individual. For example, in a claims database, the SSN for the primary subscriber may also be used for the subscriber's spouse and/or children. However, using prior work in information theory, researchers have the means to estimate the discriminatory power of the available identifiers and the chances of uniquely identifying an individual within a single dataset or across multiple datasets.

The discriminatory power of a given identifier or set of identifiers can be quantified using the Shannon entropy. This is calculated as the sum of the absolute value (abs) of ($p*\log_2(p)$), where p is the proportion of records captured by each unique value of that identifier or set of identifiers.[41] Assume that you have a simple dataset of one variable (sex) and three records, one male and two females. In this scenario, the discriminatory power of the variable, sex, is equal to abs$((0.33)*(\log_2*0.33))$ + abs$((0.67)*(\log_2*0.67))$ = 0.92. Using this method, the discriminatory power of each available identifier or set of identifiers can be measured, and identifiers or sets of identifiers can be ranked from most to least discriminatory. Notice that two variables with the same number of unique values can have varying levels of discriminatory power, depending on the distribution of unique values across the records.

Additional work has led to the development of methods to assess individual identifiability or record uniqueness in a given dataset.[42,43] These methods examine the frequency distributions for every possible combination of variables in the dataset. Those variables with the highest number of unique categories and those variable combinations that identify records uniquely have the best chance of accurately identifying the entity that the information represents. For the purposes of record linkage, the minimum set of variables needed to successfully link two or more datasets is that combination of variables for which each record is identified uniquely (the mean number of records in each pocket is ~1.00).[42] Based on this guideline, researchers can request that each of the data vendors examine the percentage of unique records in their dataset identified by each combination of variables available for release. Variable combinations that approach the threshold of ~1.00 record per pocket in both of the datasets to be linked are likely to succeed. The ~1.00 threshold can be relaxed for researchers engaged in exploratory research. Researchers testing hypotheses are advised to adhere to the ~1.00 threshold, as false positives and false negatives will likely add bias to subsequent statistical analyses. SAS code for assessing record uniqueness in a dataset has been provided by Tiefu Shen and can be found at www.naaccr.org/Research/DataAnalysisTools.aspx under "Record Uniqueness."

Cook and colleagues have developed a method to determine whether more sophisticated methods, such as the probabilistic techniques that will be discussed in Chapter 4, can be used to link the given data sources.[44] This method determines the level of discriminatory power needed to link two records with a certain desired degree of confidence (e.g., 95%) by comparing the combined discriminatory power (assessed as weights) over all available variables with the difference between the current weight and the desired weight. This method is discussed in detail in Chapter 4. Briefly, it allows researchers to set a threshold for the discriminatory power needed to successfully match files (an information threshold) while meeting a prespecified false-positive rate. Once this information threshold is met, researchers should seek the minimum discriminatory power needed in order to avoid paying for more information than is required or unnecessarily compromising subject confidentiality.

Knowing how much discriminatory power is contained in each data source and the number of overlapping identifiers available allows the researcher to determine whether linkage is possible and informs future decisions regarding the minimal set of identifiers required to assure a high-quality linkage. However, establishing feasibility is not merely an issue of whether common variables exist, but also how much overlap exists for the data sources in both content and temporality.

Regarding content overlap, two datasets may have similar variables but very different approaches for coding data or handling missing data that could influence the quality of the data linkage. For example, assume that one dataset codes missing variables as "." and the second dataset codes missing variables using interpolated values. While it is possible to establish a mechanical record link in this setting, the linked data may not provide useful information or, worse, may be misleading. As another example, assume that researchers are linking health plan claims data and electronic medical record data from two sources in an attempt to more fully capture information on vaccine receipt. Assume also that each data source has a variable called "VACCINE." If one source uses a "1" to indicate a vaccine was given and another source uses a date to indicate when the vaccine was given, researchers may find that the information they hoped to gain through the linkage is fundamentally flawed and cannot be used reliably. Thus, it is important for researchers to understand not only that a variable exists, but also the metadata related to that variable, including how and why it was captured in that form.

Researchers often wish to link data sources that are refreshed, updated, or captured on different cycles. These situations with temporally changing data pose challenges due to dynamic changes in key linkage variables. For example, addresses, phone numbers, and names (e.g., of people who marry or divorce) change over time. If this information is collected at different times for different data sources, linkage success may be diminished. Additionally, temporal disparity between datasets would affect the functional data linkage utility but may be undetected in the mechanical linkage processes. For example, if record sets are linked from sources having different collection timeframes, it may be possible to correctly link the databases mechanically, but the information from the sources will not be synchronized. This could lead to misinterpretation of the joint data patterns in the merged data. Temporal disparities in data collection could also result in mechanical link failure, since the reference variables can change for any individual over fairly short time intervals. This is an important consideration both for the evaluation of variable overlap and, ultimately, for the appropriateness of inferences made using the linked data.

Purpose and Conditions for Original Data Collection

With the evolution of data linkage techniques, researchers are now able to link multiple sources of data, including administrative health plan claims, disease registries, cohort studies, electronic medical records, financial data, and environmental data. In addition to confirming that data sources can be linked from a technical aspect, researchers must also consider ethical and legal restrictions that may limit the use of each data source that the investigator wishes to link. Two hypothetical scenarios are provided below.

Scenario 1: A researcher wishes to link State cancer registry data to administrative health plan claims data from a private health insurer to determine the impact of provider characteristics on the likelihood of a patient receiving a particular treatment. However, the insurer will not release provider information due to privacy agreements in place between the insurance company and physicians.

Scenario 2: A researcher wishes to link cohort data (previously collected in a prospective cohort study) to administrative health plan claims to evaluate the rate of sexually transmitted diseases or mental health conditions for people who participated in the cohort study. As part of the original study agreements, patients in a cohort study were told that potentially sensitive health information (e.g., treatment for sexually transmitted disease, treatment for severe mental illness) would not be collected or used as part of the research.

These hypothetical scenarios are presented to demonstrate the importance of understanding the original purposes for the data sources that the researcher hopes to use for data linkage, including limitations or conditions for data use that might affect the proposed research. Investing the time to ensure that the research objectives can be met without negative consequences for involved parties is an important step in assessing the feasibility of data linkage.

Ownership of Data

In addition to practical and ethical considerations, described above, determining ownership of data and restrictions on data use are necessary steps for researchers who want to link data. First, identifying the "owner" of each data source will ensure that the ethical and practical considerations noted above can be addressed in the research-planning phase. Next, the researcher can begin to outline a data-governance process to ensure that the original data owners are informed of and approve the use of their data for the study in question as well as any subsequent uses of the resulting linked dataset. Generally, the data-governance plan should define:

- **Who** owns the data, who must grant approval for data use, and who may be granted access to the data.
- **What** regulatory requirements the data are subject to and what is considered "acceptable use" of the data. For example, it is possible that the data, when linked, will be subject to additional regulatory requirements not pertinent to the original unlinked data.
- **Where** the data will reside.
- **When** the various stakeholders identified above are brought in to the governance process. For example, are there requirements for original data owners to review and approve manuscripts before submission for publication in a peer-reviewed journal?
- **How** data use approvals will be granted and how the data will be managed and secured.
- **Why** the data are to be linked. What are the overarching purpose behind and goal for this linkage?

Proactive development of a data-governance process provides several benefits to the researcher. First, it will help identify before study initiation potential limits on use and publication of the data. Data vendors with little experience working with academic researchers may require more information regarding the publication process before defining data use limits. Additionally, governance definition will inform the security infrastructure development and risk-management planning discussed in Chapter 2 by identifying who will have access to the data, where data will reside, and how data will be managed. Finally, a well-defined and consistently enforced data-governance process will demonstrate to potential data owners that the researcher is committed to acting as a "good steward" of the data and building a relationship as a trusted partner to the data vendor.

The data governance process will both inform and be informed by the nature of the Data Use Agreements (DUAs) between the researcher and data partner and the applicable regulatory requirements. Proactive planning when developing the DUA will allow the researcher and data partner to identify and discuss the parameters for all potential uses of the data, including whether to allow for future linking to additional datasets and whether and when the data partner will require review and approval of resulting research products (e.g., manuscripts, abstracts). Particularly important for academic researchers, these agreements may limit publication of findings; it is important that negotiations take place early in the data-governance process to ensure that dissemination of evidence is not limited and that expectations of the original data owner and the researcher are clearly outlined.

The governance process should likewise document the nature and extent of the required Institutional Review Board (IRB) review. Large multisite studies will require a higher level of coordination among IRBs. Researchers with such studies are strongly advised to consider centralized or federated IRB structures. The vast majority of individual linking projects, however, will require review by only a single IRB. Researchers intending to produce a linked dataset for use in multiple studies, whether single or multisite, should strongly consider developing and seeking IRB approval of an "umbrella" protocol. This protocol would "cover the establishment of the research database, including information on items like data processing and governance."[45] The umbrella protocol can be amended to incorporate subsequent studies, if necessary, or subsequent studies can submit separate IRB protocols referencing the umbrella protocol.

Data Sharing and Security Concerns

As mentioned above, a well-defined and consistently enforced data-governance process demonstrates the researcher's desire to be a trusted partner to data vendors and others who manage large datasets. Critical to establishing and maintaining this relationship are documented processes and procedures for securing identifiable information.

Adequate planning to protect identifiable information is crucial to receiving authority to move forward with studies that otherwise may not be allowed. We provide guidance in Chapter 2 for researchers who are building their own security systems. However, not all researchers have the resources available to build such systems. In addition, not all data partners/vendors are comfortable with releasing private health information or patient-level identifiers to researchers. There are several options available to researchers who wish to link data sources but who encounter resource limitations or who are unable to negotiate successfully for access to a partner's data. In such cases, researchers should work with data partners/vendors to determine whether hash encryption, third-party linkage, and honest brokers would satisfy security needs to allow the project to move forward.

When existing identifiers may not be released or transmitted, records can be linked effectively using identifiers encrypted before original data holder release using cryptographic hash functions.[46,47] An example is the National Security Agency's Secure Hash Algorithm v2 (SHA-2), published by the National Institute of Standards and Technology.[48] SHA-2 values cannot be reverse engineered and are widely used in security applications. Applications typically include formatting the input and concatenating a prefix, one or more variables, and a postfix. Formatting these data elements identically and applying the SHA-2 algorithm using the same key will generate the same encrypted identifier in each dataset, which can be linked deterministically to other datasets that use the same formatting, data elements, and key. Actual identifiers may be stripped and the datasets still merged, allowing data partners to limit any risks related to transferring data with Protected Health Information (PHI) for research purposes.

Another option is to involve a third-party vendor or honest broker to act as an independent source for managing data. Third-party vendors typically have extensive experience managing PHI and securing data, which can be reassuring for vendors who are wary of transferring data to researchers. Honest brokers provide a "firewall" between clinical or private health data and researchers. Individuals identified as honest brokers or third-party vendors are generally selected to ensure the privacy of data and to minimize any conflicts of interest that could exist.[49] One note of caution is that encryption through vendors is generally limited to exact matching. Thus, strict coordination of efforts for standardizing variables before encryption becomes critical. If the project is able to determine an effective group of variables to link on and the effective standardization of all the variables, then these algorithms can be applied at the data custodian site before encryption. A good practice would be to share SAS code with all data custodians that can run the code on the original data onsite. Then only the encrypted identifiers need to be released, and the link is done on the encrypted identifier using the deterministic approach. This will result in identical results as would be obtained from having access to the full identifiers due to the mathematical properties of these hash functions.[46,47] It should be noted, however, that the difficulty of using a third party for data linkage will be in determining the linkage approach (determining the matching variables and standardization) without interacting with the data or having the opportunity to do validation checks of the match results.

Methods for Privacy Protection in Record Linkage

In practice, you can limit exposure of Personally Identifiable Information by making available a small representative sample of the data, building the linkage algorithm iteratively with the sample, then sharing the SAS code, to then receive the full data with only the encrypted IDs.

Interacting with the identifiers to refine the linkage approach and validating the results are important to obtain high-quality record linkage. Recently, for most data operations, differential privacy has become the norm for privacy protection.[50] However, privacy in record linkage is fundamentally different from most other data operations; it is difficult to tackle because the goal of record linkage is to exactly identify the real-world entity represented by the data so that the linkage can be made accurately even among twins and family members. Privacy, defined as protecting the identity of patients included in the data source, is in direct conflict with the goals of record linkage. Nonetheless, it is important to note that the information that needs most protection is the sensitive health information rather than the identity information. Removing identifying information from the sensitive health information will adequately protect the confidentiality of the health information without interfering with accurate linkage. Because of this, we must distinguish between identity disclosure (Who is this person?) and sensitive attribute disclosure (Does this person have cancer?). Identity disclosure has little potential for harm on its own. The sensitive attribute disclosure is where confidentiality can be breached.[51-55]

Kum and colleagues have proposed a new approach for Privacy Preserving Interactive Record Linkage (PPIRL), which defines the privacy goal as a guarantee against attribute disclosure while minimizing identity disclosure. The usability goal is to determine the minimum amount of information required while interacting with the data for high-quality record linkage and to release only that information.[52,54] PPIRL is a framework that can be deployed in a record linkage project to reduce the risk of sensitive attribute disclosure by using a combination of approaches: (1) decoupling data using newly generated encrypted identifiers, or pseudonyms (discussed in Chapter 2); (2) adding fake data to block against group disclosure (i.e., by temporarily adding fake people without cancer to the registry so that one cannot infer with confidence that an identified subject has cancer merely by their being on the registry); and (3) restricting information in any variable by limiting it to what is needed (e.g., using Soundex of name).

Selection of privacy protection methods in record linkage is a separate decision to the approach selected for doing the record linkage (deterministic or probabilistic). One-way hash encryption can support any deterministic methods and give identical results. PPIRL can support both deterministic and probabilistic methods and allows for interaction with the data for iteratively refining the linkage method and validating the results. Thus, results will not differ from those from other described methods for implementing the data linkage methods selected. However, PPIRL may provide better protection of patient privacy in settings where confidentiality concerns are of paramount importance.

Building the Team

A "team science" approach is required to successfully develop and execute a linking project. This involves multidisciplinary collaborations in which experts from different fields share insights, perspectives, and tools from their respective disciplines. These individuals need to be technical experts but also must be able to bridge technical and disciplinary gaps and communicate effectively across the team to achieve a cohesive solution.[56] However, true "team science" must be "transdisciplinary," defined as integrating the disciplines within the research framework in a way that moves the project beyond what would be achieved by any of the individual disciplines alone.[57,58] Linking data effectively requires identifying individuals from diverse fields, including population science, information science and technology, [bio]statistics/analytics, and regulatory/legal project management. It is important to identify and recruit potential team members in the early stages of the linkage project because each will have important and specific insight regarding feasibility.

Chapter 4. An Overview of Record Linkage Methods

Overview

Randomized controlled trials (RCTs) remain the gold standard for assessing intervention efficacy; however, RCTs are not always feasible or sufficiently timely. Perhaps more importantly, RCT results often cannot be generalized due to a lack of inclusion of "real-world" combinations of interventions and heterogeneous patients.[1-4] With recent advances in information technology, data, and statistical methods, there is tremendous promise in leveraging ever-growing repositories of secondary data to support comparative effectiveness and public health research.[2,6,39] While there are many advantages to using these secondary data sources, they are often limited in scope, which in turn limits their utility in addressing important questions in a comprehensive manner. These limitations can be overcome by linking data from multiple sources such as health registries and administrative claims data.[7,14-16]

An extensive and complex process, record linkage is both a science and an art.[59] While the process can be difficult to navigate, many effective strategies have been developed and documented in the health services literature. However, new policies and concerns over data security are making it more challenging for investigators to link data using traditional methods. Of particular importance are increasingly restrictive policies governing Protected Health Information that severely limit access to the unique identifiers on which many documented strategies rely. In light of these challenges, there is a need to increase understanding and extend capacity to perform reliable linkages in varying scenarios of data availability.

In this chapter, we guide the reader through an overview of data linkage methods and discuss the strengths and weaknesses of various linkage strategies in the effort to develop and document a set of best practices for conducting data linkages with optimal validity and reliability, and minimal risk to privacy and confidentiality.

Data Cleaning and Standardization

Data come in different shapes, sizes, and quality, creating scenarios that must be considered in building a linkage algorithm. For instance, demographic information often contains typographical and data entry errors, such as transposed Social Security Number (SSN) digits and misspellings. An individual's information sometimes changes over time, with life changes such as marriage or moving leading to changes in one's name or address. People sometimes deliberately report false information to defraud insurance providers or to avoid detection. Twins can have very similar information. Finally, the spouses and/or children of the family's primary health insurance subscriber sometimes use the primary subscriber's information. These idiosyncrasies are what make data linkage difficult, so the more work done upfront to clean and standardize the data, the better the chances of a successful linkage.

With this in mind, the first step after data delivery is to examine the nature of the data, paying particular attention to the way information is stored, the completeness of the identifying information, the extent to

which information overlaps, and the presence of any idiosyncrasies in the data. By doing so, steps can be taken to clean and standardize the available information across data sources to minimize false matches attributable to typographical errors. Table 4.1 shows some of the commonly seen issues to clean, account for, and/or standardize before beginning the linkage process.

Many data manipulation techniques are available in commonly used software (e.g., SAS and Stata) to facilitate the data cleaning and standardization process. Using these techniques renders all linkage variables the same across data sources—that is, variables that will be compared are forced into the same case (e.g., all uppercase), the same format (e.g., 01SEP2013), the same content (e.g., stripped of all punctuation and digits), and the same length.

Additionally, identifiers can be parsed into separate pieces of information. For instance, full names can be parsed into first, middle, last, and maiden names; dates of birth can be parsed into month, day, and year of birth; and addresses can be parsed into street, city, State, and ZIP Code. Parsing identifiers into separate pieces where possible allows the researcher to maximize the amount of available information and give credit for partial agreement when record pairs do not agree character for character. This is particularly important in accounting for changes across time, such as a name change after marriage or an address change after a move. In such cases, matching on the separate pieces allows for the possibility of partial credit that, when combined with other information, may provide sufficient evidence that the records being compared represent the same person.

Table 4.1. Common variations found in selected linkage identifiers

Field	Type	Examples
Names	Case	John Smith	JOHN SMITH
	Nicknames	Charles	Chuck
	Synonyms	William	Bill
	Prefixes	Dr. John Smith
	Suffixes	John Smith, III
	Punctuation	O'Malley	Smith-Taylor	Smith, Jr.
	Spaces	John Smith, Jr
	Digits	J2ohn Smith
	Initials	AM	A.M.	Anne Marie
	Transposition	John Smith	Smith John
Address	Abbreviations	RD	Road	DR	Drive
Dates	Format	01012013	01-01-2013	01JAN2013
	Invalid values	Month = 13	Day = 32	Birth year = 2025	Date = 29FEB2013
Social Security Number	Format	999999999	999-99-9999	999 99 9999
Geographic locations	Abbreviations	NC	North Carolina
	FIPS codes	North Carolina = 37
	SSA codes	North Carolina = 34
	ZIP Codes	99999	99999-9999
	Concatenation of State and county codes	Mecklenburg County, NC	37119
Sex	Format	Male / Female	M / F	1 / 2

FIPS = Federal Information Processing Standards; SSA = Social Security Administration.

Chapter 4. An Overview of Record Linkage Methods

Other techniques have been developed to account for minor misspellings and typographical errors. Here are three examples.

1. Strings can be converted to phonetic codes (e.g., Soundex or New York State Immunization Information System) before comparison.
2. Strings can be compared using editing distance techniques to determine how many steps (insertions, deletions, transpositions, etc.) are required to get from String A to String B. For example, it would require one step—one character deletion—to get from "Billy" to "Bill."
3. Names can be linked to an array of synonyms (e.g., "William" and "Bill") to account for the use of nicknames.[60-62]

Each of these techniques has been shown to improve the accuracy of string comparisons.[61,62] In Appendix 4.1 we have provided sample SAS code for performing these functions.

Finally, it is important to consider informational overlap in the available linkage identifiers. As in statistical modeling, where two strongly correlated variables should not be included together in the model, variables with overlapping information should not be included in the same linkage algorithm. In such cases, assigning credit for matches on both variables (e.g., ZIP Code and county) is redundant, leading to an overestimate of the extent to which two records agree. Similarly, assigning separate penalties for nonmatches on overlapping variables (e.g., first name and first name initial) is redundant, leading to an overestimate of the extent to which two records disagree. In the case of overlapping variables, researchers can pick either one or take the most informative match; for example, if two records match on ZIP Code and county, then the match on ZIP Code is more informative.

Alternatively, if there are concerns regarding the quality of two overlapping variables, the researcher may wish to explore the use of both variables to improve match rates. For example, if county to county matches are made but ZIP is off by one digit due to a typo, the researcher may choose to confirm the match based on the county variable. This redundancy in information can be used to account for random errors, if used properly. The researcher must weigh the extent to which the inclusion of additional variables is thought to improve the match (without resulting in additional false matches). Similarly, the researcher may also desire to retain overlapping variables to perform iterative deterministic matching (match first on ZIP Code for exact matches and then on county when ZIP Codes do not match exactly).

How much data cleaning and standardization are necessary depends on the quality of the data, the research question, and the discretion of the researcher. While cleaning can improve linkage rates, the cleaning process can be quite labor intensive, so researchers should consider the cost-benefit analysis before investing a significant amount of time on cleaning the data. Cleaning has been highly recommended if the data quality is poor and/or only a few identifiers are available.[63] When the data quality is relatively good or many identifiers are available to override the errors, the cost usually outweighs the reward.[64] The scope of the project should be considered as well. If the project is exploratory in nature, then the potential harm of false positives and false negatives may be negligible. Conversely, a hypothesis test may be significantly biased by false positives and false negatives.[65] Each of these considerations should be weighed against one another in the effort to determine whether data cleaning is prudent.

Linkage Methods

There are two main types of linkage algorithms: deterministic and probabilistic. Both have been successfully implemented in previous research studies.[11,21,24,35,36,44,59,66-80] Choosing the best algorithm to use in a given situation depends on many interacting factors, such as time; resources; the research question; and the quantity and quality of the variables available to link, including the degree to which they individually and collectively are able to identify an individual uniquely. With this in mind, it is important that researchers be equipped with data linkage algorithms for varying scenarios. The key is to develop algorithms to extract and make use of enough meaningful information to make sound decisions. In this section, we will review the main algorithm types and discuss the strengths and weaknesses of each in an effort to derive a set of guidelines describing which algorithms are best in varying scenarios of data availability, data quality, and investigator goals.

Deterministic Linkage Methods

Deterministic algorithms determine whether record pairs agree or disagree on a given set of identifiers, where agreement on a given identifier is assessed as a discrete—"all-or-nothing"—outcome. Match status can be assessed in a single step or in multiple steps. In a single-step strategy, records are compared all at once on the full set of identifiers. A record pair is classified as a match if the two records agree, character for character, on all identifiers and the record pair is uniquely identified (no other record pair matched on the same set of values). A record pair is classified as a nonmatch if the two records disagree on any of the identifiers or if the record pair is not uniquely identified. In a multiple-step strategy (also referred to as an iterative or stepwise strategy), records are matched in a series of progressively less restrictive steps in which record pairs that do not meet a first round of match criteria are passed to a second round of match criteria for further comparison. If a record pair meets the criteria in any step, it is classified as a match. Otherwise, it is classified as a nonmatch. These two approaches to deterministic linkage can also be called "exact deterministic" (requiring an exact match on all identifiers) and "approximate or iterative deterministic" (requiring an exact match on one of several rounds of matching but not on all possible identifiers).

While the existence of a gold standard in registry-to-claims linkages is a matter of debate, the iterative deterministic approach employed by the National Cancer Institute to create the SEER (Surveillance, Epidemiology and End Results)-Medicare linked dataset[81,82] has demonstrated high validity and reliability and has been employed successfully in multiple updates of the SEER-Medicare linked dataset.[83,84] The algorithm consists of a sequence of deterministic matches using different match criteria in each successive round.

In the first step, two records must match on SSN and one of the following:

- First and last name (allowing for fuzzy matches, such as nicknames)
- Last name, month of birth, and sex
- First name, month of birth, and sex

If SSN is missing or does not match, or two records fail to meet the initial match criteria, they may be declared a match if they agree on the match criteria in a second round of deterministic linkages, in which two records must match on last name, first name, month of birth, sex, and one of the following:

- Seven to eight digits of the SSN
- Two or more of the following: year of birth, day of birth, middle initial, or date of death

In situations in which full identifiers or partial identifiers are available but may not be released or transmitted, a deterministic linkage on encrypted identifiers may be employed. Quantin and colleagues[33,46-47] have developed procedures for encrypting identifiers using cryptographic hash functions so identifiers needed for linkage can be released directly to researchers without compromising patient confidentiality. A cryptographic hash function, such as the Secure Hash Algorithm version 2 (SHA-2), released by the National Security Agency and published by the National Institute of Standards and Technology, is a deterministic procedure that takes input and returns an output that was intentionally changed by an algorithm. Due to its deterministic attributes and the inability to reverse-engineer a hashed value, it has been widely adopted for security applications and procedures. Quantin's research shows that records can successfully be linked via deterministic algorithms using identifiers encrypted before release.[46,85-86] It should be noted, however, that record pairs matched on encrypted identifiers cannot be manually reviewed or validated.

Probabilistic Linkage Methods

The deterministic approach ignores the fact that certain identifiers or certain values have more discriminatory power than others do. Probabilistic strategies have been developed to assess (1) the discriminatory power of each identifier and (2) the likelihood that two records are a true match based on whether they agree or disagree on the various identifiers.

According to the model developed by Fellegi and Sunter,[33] matched record pairs can be designated as matches, possible matches, or nonmatches based on the calculation of linkage scores and the application of decision rules. Say we have two files, A and B, where file A contains 100 records and File B contains 1,000 records. The comparison space is the Cartesian product made up of all possible record pairs (A * B), or 100 * 1,000 = 100,000 possible matches. Each pair in the comparison space is either a true match or a true nonmatch.

When dealing with large files (e.g., claims files), considering the entire Cartesian product is often computationally impractical. In these situations, it is advisable to reduce the comparison space to only those matched pairs that meet certain basic criteria. This is referred to as "blocking," which serves to functionally subset a large dataset into a smaller dataset of individuals with at least one common characteristic, such as geographic region or a specific clinical condition. For instance, the number of matched pairs to be considered may be limited to only those matched pairs that agree on clinical diagnosis or on both month of birth and county of residence. Those record pairs that do not meet the matching criteria specified in the blocking phase are automatically classified as nonmatches and removed from consideration. To account for true matches that were not blocked together (due to data issues), typically multiple passes are used so that rows that were not blocked together in one pass have the potential to be blocked and compared in another pass to avoid automatic misclassification. Since two records cannot be matched on missing information, the variables chosen for the blocking phase should be relatively complete, having few missing values. Blocking strategies such as this reduce the set of potential matches to a more manageable number. Because blocking strategies can influence linkage success, Christen and Goiser recommend that researchers report the specific steps of their blocking strategy.[87]

The two records in every matched pair identified in the blocking phase are compared on each linkage identifier, producing an agreement pattern. The weight assigned to agreement or disagreement on each identifier is assessed as a likelihood ratio, comparing the probability that true matches agree on the identifier ("m-probability") to the probability that false matches randomly agree on the identifier ("u-probability").

The m-probability can be estimated based on values reported in published linkage literature or by taking a random sample of pairs from the comparison space, assigning match status via manual review, and calculating the probability that two records agree on a particular identifier when they are true matches. The u-probability can be calculated by observing the probability that two records agree on a particular identifier merely by chance; for example, the u-probability for month of birth is 1/12, or .083. Calculating value-specific u-probabilities for an identifier based on the frequency of each value and the likelihood that two records would agree on a given value simply by chance yields additional information.

For instance, a match on a rare surname such as Lebowski is less likely to occur by chance, and is thereby assigned greater weight than a match on a common surname such as Smith. This principle can be applied to any linkage identifier for which values are differentially distributed.

When two records agree on an identifier, an agreement weight is calculated by dividing the m-probability by the u-probability and taking the $\log_2$ of the quotient. For example, if the probability that true matches agree on month of birth is 97 percent and the probability that false matches randomly agree on month of birth is 8.3 percent (1/12), then the agreement weight for month of birth would be calculated as ($\log_2[.97/.083]$), or 3.54. When two records disagree on an identifier, a disagreement weight is calculated by dividing 1 minus the m-probability by 1 minus the u-probability. For example, the disagreement weight for month of birth would be calculated as ($\log_2 [(1-.97)/(1-.083)]$), or -4.93.

While the method above accounts for the discriminatory power of the identifier, it does not yet take into account the *degree* to which records agree on a given identifier. This is important for fields where typographical errors are likely to occur (e.g., names, addresses). Assigning *partial agreement weights* in situations where two strings do not match character for character can account for minor typographical errors, including spelling errors in names or transposed digits in dates or SSNs.[60-62] Partial agreement weights for string comparators can account for both the length of the string and common human errors made in alphanumeric strings. If all of the characters in a string are matched character by character across two files, then the agreement weight is maximized (set at the full agreement weight). If there are no characters in common, where common characters are defined by Winkler as being no further than ($[m/2] - 1$) where m = (max [length of string in file 1, length of string in file 2]), then the agreement weight is zero.[62] String comparator values take into account characteristics that would reduce the likelihood of matching, such as string length, number of transpositions of characters, number of characters in common, and location on the string where the nonmatch occurs. For example, lower weights would be assigned for short names or when the first characters of the string are not matched between the two files. From Winkler's prior example, larger string comparator values were assigned when comparing "Shack**le**ford" and "Shack**el**ford" (string comparator value = 0.9848) than "**L**ampley" and "**C**ampley" (string comparator value = 0.9048). The full agreement weight for the identifier can then be multiplied by the string comparator value to generate a partial agreement weight. For example, if the full agreement weight for first name is 12 and the string comparator value is 0.95 that the first name on one record matches the first name on another record, then the partial agreement weight would be equal to 12*0.95, or 11.4. Once the weights, full and partial, for each identifier have been calculated, the linkage score for each matched pair is equal to the sum of the weights across all linkage identifiers. Use of string comparator methods may significantly improve match rates if a large number of typographical errors are expected.

An initial assessment of linkage quality can be gained by plotting the match scores in a histogram. If the linkage algorithm is working properly, then the plot should show a bimodal distribution of scores, with one large peak among the lower scores for the large proportion of likely nonmatches and a second smaller peak among the higher scores for the smaller set of likely matches. The cutoff threshold for match/nonmatch status will be a score somewhere in the trough between the two peaks. Depending on the research question and the nature of the study, the initial threshold can be adjusted to be more conservative (higher score) or more liberal (lower score). A more conservative threshold will maximize the specificity of the linkage decision, as only those record pairs with a high score will be counted as matches. Conversely, a more liberal threshold will maximize the sensitivity of the linkage decision to possible matches.

Cook and colleagues[44] define the cutoff threshold as the difference between the desired weight and the starting weight. Given two files, A and B, the starting weight for each record pair is equal to the $\log_2$ of the odds of picking a true match by chance,

$$\log2(E / ((A \times B) - E)),$$

where E is the number of expected matches, A is the number of records in File A, and B is the number of records in File B. If the number of records in File A is 1,000, the number of records in File B is 1,000,000, and the expected number of matches is 10 percent of 1,000 records in File A, or 100, then the starting weight will be -23.25. The "expected" number of matches can be determined by prior research, prior knowledge, or an educated guess if there is no precedent.

If P is the desired probability that two records were not matched together by chance (i.e., the desired positive predictive value), then the desired weight for each record pair is equal to the log2 of the odds associated with P:

$$\log_2(P / (1 - P)).$$

If the desired value of P is 0.95, then the desired weight is $\log_2(0.95 / (1 - 0.95)) = 4.25$. The cutoff threshold, or score needed to have a false-match rate of <0.05, is the difference between the desired weight, 4.25, and the starting weight, -23.25, which is 27.50. If the computed linkage score is greater than or equal to the cutoff threshold, then the record pair is classified as a match. If the computed linkage score is less than the cutoff threshold, then the record pair is classified as a nonmatch. Researchers wishing to maximize the sensitivity of the algorithm to potential matches can relax this threshold somewhat and manually review all record pairs with scores near the calculated cutoff.

Once this process is complete, a sample of the match decisions made by the linkage algorithm should be reviewed to ensure that the algorithm performed as intended. By reviewing match decisions, you can often identify conditions in which the algorithm could use some tweaking to account for difficult cases. For instance, frequently the children and/or spouses of the primary subscriber use the primary subscriber's SSN, thereby making it difficult to identify them as unique individuals given the large weight often assigned to agreement on SSN. Twins are another difficult case, as they have the same birthdate, frequently have similar names, and often have SSNs that differ on only one to two digits. Records for a married woman can sometimes be difficult to match when marriage leads to changes in the woman's last name and/or address. Finally, tweaks to the algorithm can often improve the performance of the algorithm on the "fuzzy" or borderline cases. By reviewing a sample of match decisions, you can tweak your algorithm to account for each of these cases, thereby improving the performance of the algorithm. This will be particularly important for researchers who hope to reuse the algorithm for future linkages (e.g., matching a new year of registry cases to a new year of administrative claims data). A summary of steps for performing probabilistic record linkage is provided below.

Summary of Steps for Probabilistic Record Linkage:

1. Estimate the *m* and *u* probabilities for each linking variable using the observed frequency of agreement and disagreement patterns among all pairs, commonly generated using the EM (expectation-maximization) algorithm described by Fellegi-Sunter.

2. Calculate agreement and disagreement weights using the m and u probabilities.

3. Calculate a total linking weight for each pair by summing the individual linking weights for each linkage variable.

4. Compare the total linkage weight to a threshold above which pairs are considered a link. The threshold is set using information generated in step 1.

Alternative Linkage Methods

The methods presented above are those most commonly used in registry-to-claims linkages. Other methods are available for researchers who have more challenging linkage scenarios. The EM algorithm[61,62] is an iterative approach to estimating m- and u-probabilities. According to Winkler, the EM algorithm provides very accurate estimates of m- and u-probabilities in situations where the amount of typographical error in the identifiers is minimal, but performs poorly when the identifiers contain numerous typographical errors. In the sorted-neighborhood approach,[88] the data sources are stacked and sorted by various combinations of the available identifiers. For each sort, all records within a window of n-records are compared. The Bayesian approach[89] is an alternative to the frequentist approach presented above. The computer science literature also includes distance-based techniques[90] as well as unsupervised and supervised machine-learning approaches.[91,92]

Selecting a Linkage Method

What kind of linkage method to employ in a given situation depends on a variety of factors, some of which are scientific and some of which are more subjective. In information-rich scenarios where direct identifiers are available and of good quality, deterministic methods have been recommended.[42] In these scenarios, deterministic methods are easy to implement, easy to interpret, and effective. In scenarios that are information poor (where direct identifiers are unavailable) and/or the data are of poor quality, probabilistic methods consistently outperform deterministic methods and thus merit the extra time and resources required to implement them. Beyond these broad guidelines, the decision is left to the researchers and their goals for the project. Herein lies the "art" of record linkage.[59] For instance, researchers studying a rare disease may want to employ probabilistic methods even in information-rich scenarios in the effort to identify every possible match and maximize sample size. Ultimately, every researcher must weigh the pros and cons of the available methods in the context of the project and choose the method that best fits the budget, timeline, allotted resources, and research question.

Evaluating Linkage Algorithms

In record linkage, there are two types of accuracy errors. A Type I error occurs when a true nonmatch is classified as a match. A Type II error occurs when a true match is classified as a nonmatch. Minimizing these errors is critical, particularly when the product will be used in a cohort study,[65] where linkage error can introduce bias into analyses. In the health sciences literature, the four metrics most often used to evaluate the accuracy of a linkage algorithm are: (1) sensitivity, (2) specificity, (3) positive predictive value, and (4) negative predictive value. Table 4.2 shows all possible outcomes of a linkage decision.

Table 4.2. True match status by algorithm output

		Algorithm Output	
		Match	Nonmatch
True Match Status	Match	A	B
	Nonmatch	C	D

"A" represents all true matches that are correctly classified as matches; "B" represents all true matches that are incorrectly classified as nonmatches; "C" represents all true nonmatches that are incorrectly classified as matches; and "D" represents all true nonmatches that are correctly classified as nonmatches.

Sensitivity = A / (A + B). Sensitivity measures the ability of an algorithm to correctly classify true matches as matches.

Specificity = C / (C + D). Specificity measures the ability of an algorithm to correctly classify true nonmatches as nonmatches.

Positive predictive value (PPV) = A / (A + C). PPV represents the proportion of matched pairs classified by the algorithm as matches that are true matches.

Negative predictive value (NPV) = D / (B + D). NPV represents the proportion of matched pairs classified by the algorithm as nonmatches that are true nonmatches.

These metrics measure an algorithm's ability to classify correctly true matches as matches, and true nonmatches as nonmatches.

Due to the large number of potential matches identified during the blocking phase, the bulk of the comparison space will be made up of true nonmatches. For this reason, Christen and Goiser[87] argue that linkage metrics that include true nonmatches (e.g., specificity and NPV) in the equation will be skewed. Instead, they recommend metrics such as the *f-measure*,[92] which represents the harmonic mean of the sensitivity, and PPV, which is not influenced by the large number of true nonmatches. The f-measure is calculated as

$$((\beta^2 + 1.0) * \text{Sensitivity} * \text{PPV}) / (\beta^2 * \text{Sensitivity} + \text{PPV}),$$

where β is equal to the user-assigned relative importance of sensitivity over PPV. If the user wishes to assign equal weight to sensitivity and PPV, then $\beta = 1.0$. If the user wishes to assign sensitivity twice the weight of PPV, then $\beta = 2.0$.

These metrics represent tradeoffs between sensitivity and specificity. Investigators hoping to maximize sensitivity may increase their false-positive rate, subsequently resulting in a smaller PPV. Those wishing to maximize specificity may increase their false-negative rate. If the goals of the investigation are to estimate all or most true cases, then investigators may want to focus on sensitivity. Otherwise, if the goals are to reduce the likelihood of including false positives, the researcher may focus on specificity. While there is no hard rule, a good linkage algorithm will typically have values of sensitivity, PPV, and the f-measure in excess of 95 percent. However, what is acceptable depends on the context of the study. If the study involves the testing of hypotheses and/or the results will have significant practical implications (e.g., findings will be incorporated into clinical practice or influence policy), a higher percent match is more desirable. On the other hand, if a study is exploratory, a lower percent match may be acceptable. What is acceptable may also vary depending on the frequency of the outcome. Researchers studying a rare disease may seek to emphasize sensitivity to maximize the sample size, while a researcher studying a more frequently occurring disease may want to emphasize PPV to ensure that matches identified by the algorithm are true matches.

Validating Linkage Results

The final step of the linkage process is the validation of the match results. Initial steps for determining linkage validity are to look for ties in which multiple record pairs identified as matches by the algorithm have exactly the same set of values. For example, common names such as "Mary Smith" or "Mike Brown" are typically repeated in large datasets, and thus have multiple matches. Where possible, ties should be adjudicated by reference to additional information. If no additional information is available, then the record pairs should be classified as nonmatches. If an algorithm is successful, there will be few to no ties.

The next step is to assess the extent to which your matched sample reflects the target population. For instance, in a study linking a single State's cancer registry to Medicare administrative claims for that State, researchers may use estimates of the percentage of cancer patients age 65 and older to determine what percentage of patients in the cancer registry would be expected to be linked to the Medicare data. If estimates indicate that

60 percent of cancer patients in the State are 65 and older, then it is reasonable to expect that 60 percent of the patients in the cancer registry will be matched with Medicare. If, instead, the researcher finds that only 30 percent of patients in the cancer registry are successfully matched, this may serve as a signal that there is a problem with the matching algorithm.

While not well documented in the literature, some form of manual review is typically employed to check the results. Before starting the manual review process, a set of decision rules is developed to standardize the decision process across reviewers. Next, a random sample is drawn from the set of all potential matches identified during the blocking phase. Following the decision rules, one or more reviewers then determine whether each potential match is a match or nonmatch. Finally, the decisions documented during the manual review process are used as a gold standard against which the decisions made by the algorithm are compared, allowing for the calculation of the sensitivity, PPV, and f-measure of the algorithm. A good algorithm should have scores of 95 percent or better across the three metrics.

Final Remarks

In this chapter, we have provided an overview of data linkage methodology from the point of data delivery to the reporting of the linkage results. We noted that if data quality is good (e.g., unique identifiers with few typographical errors and/missing values), the cost of the labor-intensive process of cleaning and standardizing the data is not worth the reward, and therefore not recommended. In this scenario, deterministic linkage methods are accurate, straightforward, and easy to implement.

If data quality is poor (e.g., little identifying information and/or numerous typographical errors), cleaning and standardizing the data before linkage can greatly improve linkage rates. In these scenarios, iterative deterministic techniques or more sophisticated probabilistic techniques are recommended. Combining deterministic and probabilistic methods can improve efficiency and save computational resources. When combining methods, a deterministic match on all identifiers can be executed first to identify certain matches. The remaining record pairs that disagree on at least one of the identifiers can be submitted for probabilistic matching. Using deterministic and probabilistic methods in this stepwise fashion reduces the number of record pairs that will be processed in the more resource-intensive probabilistic matching phase.

In order to limit the computational resources required to compare the Cartesian product of all possible matches, blocking should be implemented to reduce the comparison space to record pairs that agree on some basic criteria (e.g., date of birth and county or clinical diagnosis). This process can improve computational efficiency and performance substantially. It is important to do multiple blocking passes to account for data issues on the blocking variable. Blocking techniques can have a significant effect on the linkage results, and thus researchers should report the blocking method.

Both deterministic procedures and probabilistic procedures should be considered iterative. After completing the initial linkage, a random sample of match decisions should be reviewed to ensure that the algorithm is performing as intended. If the review process reveals opportunities for improvement, then the algorithm should be adjusted to account for the identified weaknesses.

Once the linkage process is complete, the results should be compared to known metrics. For instance, if it is known that 20 percent of cancer patients in the State are covered by private insurance, then roughly 20 percent of the records in a State cancer-registry database should match to private insurance claims. If the observed match rate differs substantially from the expected results, then the linkage method should be reevaluated and repeated.

Chapter 4. An Overview of Record Linkage Methods

When reporting linkage results, estimates of the sensitivity, PPV, and f-measure of the algorithm should be reported to provide readers with a characterization of the validity and reliability of the linkage product. Due to the disproportionately large number of nonmatched pairs identified during the blocking phase, measures that include the number of nonmatched pairs in the calculation (e.g., specificity and NPV) should not be reported.

In the next chapter, we will empirically demonstrate the approaches described in this chapter and develop and test a series of deterministic and probabilistic algorithms for scenarios of varying unique identifier availability.

Researchers who wish to learn more about data linkage approaches and techniques beyond those covered in this chapter are referred to Dr. William Winkler's list of Statistical Data Editing References: http://citeseerx.ist.psu.edu/viewdoc/summary;jsessionid=BAA7B495D9CFBEB3276C67AB96BFFA6D?doi=10.1.1.79.1519.

Appendix 4.1. Useful SAS Functions and Procedures

Data Cleaning and Standardization

Remove all special characters

> **Syntax**: compress(varname, ".,'{}[]/\()+~`!@#$%^&*_<>?");
>
> **Ex**. Remove all special characters from the string "(John_Doe!)"
> newname = compress(name, ".,'{}[]/\()+~`!@#$%^&*_<>?");
> put name;
> JohnDoe

Remove a specific character

> **Syntax**: compress(varname, "-");
>
> **Ex**. Remove all dashes from the string "999-99-9999"
> newssn = compress(ssn, "-");
> put newssn;
> 999999999

Remove all punctuation

> **Syntax**: compress(varname, ,"P");
>
> **Ex**. Remove all punctuation from "O'Brien-Smith"
> newname = compress(name, ,"P");
> put newname;
> OBrienSmith

Remove all digits

> **Syntax**: compress(varname, ,"D");
>
> **Ex**. Remove all digits from the string "J2ohn"
> newname = compress(name, ,"D");
> put newname;
> John

Remove all spaces

> **Syntax**: compress(varname, " ");
>
> **Ex**. Remove all spaces from the string "Van Slyke"
> newname = compress(name, " ");
> put newname;
> VanSlyke

Remove leading and trailing spaces

> **Syntax**: strip(varname);
>
> **Ex**. Remove all leading and trailing spaces from the string " John "
> newname = strip(firstname);
> put newname;
> John

Remove extra spaces with a single space

> **Syntax**: compbl(varname);
>
> **Ex**. Remove all extra spaces from the string "Van   Slyke"
> newname = compbl(name);
> put newname;
> Van Slyke

Extracting data from a substring

> **Syntax**: substr(varname, start, count);
>
> **Ex**. Extract first initial from the name "John"
> initial = substr(name, 1, 1);
> put initial;
> J

Search for and replace a string

> **Syntax**: tranwrd(varname, string_to_be_replaced, replacement_string);
>
> **Ex**. Find all instances of the string "Road" in the string "Anystreet Road" and replace with "Rd."
> newstreet = tranwrd(street, "Road", "Rd.");
> put newstreet;
> Anystreet Rd.

Appendix 4.1. Useful SAS Functions and Procedures

Make all characters in a string uppercase

> **Syntax**: upcase(varname);
>
> **Ex**. Make all characters in the string "John" uppercase
> newname = upcase(name);
> put newname;
> JOHN

Make all characters in a string lowercase

> **Syntax**: lowcase(varname);
>
> **Ex**. Make all characters in the string "JOHN" lowercase
> newname = lowcase(name);
> put newname;
> john

Make all characters in a string proper case (1st character uppercase, remaining characters lowercase)

> **Syntax**: propcase(varname);
>
> **Ex**. Convert the string "JOHN" to proper case
> newname = propcase(name);
> put newname;
> John

Concatenate two strings

> **Syntax**: varname1||varname2;
> -OR-
> **Syntax**: cat(varname1,varname2);
>
> **Ex**. Concatenate first name ("JOHN") and last name ("DOE")
> newname = firstname||lastname;
> newname = cat(firstname, lastname);
> put newname;
> JOHNDOE
>
> For more information on CAT functions see:
> "Purrfectly fabulous feline functions" by Louise S. Hadden

Parse out pieces in a string

Syntax: scan(varname, count, delimiter);

Ex. Parse out first, middle and last name from "JOHN SMITH DOE"
firstname = scan(fullname, 1, " ");
put firstname;
JOHN

middlename = scan(fullname, 2, " ");
put middlename;
SMITH

lastname = scan(fullname, 3, " ");
put lastname;
DOE

Convert string to phonetic code

Syntax: soundex(varname);

Ex. Convert the first name "JOHN" to phonetic code
newname = soundex(firstname);
put newname;
J5

Calculate editing distance

Syntax: spedis(varname);
-OR-
Syntax: complev(varname);
-OR-
Syntax: compged(varname);

Ex. Determine the editing distance between 'CHARLES' and 'CHARLIE'
name1 = 'CHARLES';
name2 = 'CHARLIE';
spedis = spedis(name1, name2);
put spedis;
21

complev = complev(name1, name2);
put complev;
2

compged = compged(name1, name2);
put compged;
200

Note: For a comparison of the editing distance functions, see "Fuzzy Matching using the COMPGED Function" by Paulette Staum.

Appendix 4.1. Useful SAS Functions and Procedures

Social Security Number (SSN) Validation

See "Identifying Invalid Social Security Numbers" by Paulette Staum and Sally Dai in the NorthEast SAS Users Group (2007).

Variable Encryption

> **Syntax**: md5(varname);
>
> **Ex**. Encrypt the name "JOHNDOE"
> newname = md5(name);
> put newname;
> "ãiŒƒúÀ¥—q...zÅ

General Matching Techniques

Loop to determine how many SSN digits match

> attrib SSN_DIG_MATCH format = 1. label = '# of SSN Digits that Match';
> SSN_DIG_MATCH = 0;
>
> do i = 1 to 9; if substr(put(CCR_SSN,$9.),i,1) = substr(put(PAYER_SSN,$9.),i,1) then SSN_DIG_MATCH + 1;
> end;

Compare beginnings of strings, up to length of shorter string

> **Syntax**: compare(compress(string1,' '), compress(string2,' '), ':');
>
> **Ex**. Compare the last names 'WILLIAMS-SMITH' and 'WILLIAMS' character-for-character up to length of shorter name
>
> if compare(compress(lastname1,' '), compress(lastname2,' '), ':') = 0
> then ln_compare = 'match';
>
> *** Use with caution. This technique is a useful way to identify cases to manually review (e.g., names reported differently over time).

Compare ends of strings (in reverse order), up to length of shorter string

> **Syntax**: compare(compress(reverse(string1),' '), compress(reverse(string2),' '), ':');
>
> **Ex**. Compare the last names 'WILLIAMS-SMITH' and 'SMITH' character-for-character up to length of shorter name
>
> if compare(compress(reverse(lastname1),' '),
> compress(reverse(lastname2),' '), ':') = 0
> then ln_compare = 'match';
>
> *** Use with caution. This technique is a useful way to identify cases to manually review (e.g., names reported differently over time).

Surveillance, Epidemiology and End Results (SEER)-Medicare Algorithm

```
/* INITIATE SEER-MEDICARE MATCH INDICATOR */
attrib seermedicare format = 1. length = 3.;
seermedicare = 0;

/* IF SSN MATCHES */
if ssn then do;
        /* IF FIRST NAME AND LAST NAME MATCH */
        if ( firstname and lastname )
        or
        /* IF LAST NAME, MONTH OF BIRTH AND GENDER MATCH */
        (lastname and birthmonth and gender )
        or
        /* IF FIRST NAME, MONTH OF BIRTH AND GENDER MATCH */
        ( firstname and birthmonth and gender )
        then seermedicare = 1;
end;

/* IF SSN DOES NOT MATCH, AND LAST NAME, FIRST NAME, MONTH OF BIRTH */
/* AND GENDER MATCH                                                 */
if not ssn and ( lastname and firstname and birthmonth and gender )
then do;
  /* IF 7+ SSN DIGITS MATCH OR 2+ OF YEAR OF BIRTH, DAY OF BIRTH, */
  /* MIDDLE INITIAL OR DATE OF DEATH MATCH                        */
    if (ssn_dig_match >= 7) or
        (sum(of birthyear, birthday, middleinitial, deathdate) >= 2)
        then seermedicare = 1;
end;
```

Probabilistic Matching Techniques

Calculate u-probability

Ex. Generate u-probability for firstname

```
proc freq data = lib.dataset_a (keep = firstname) noprint;
table firstname / norow nocol out = lib.fnfreq;
run;

data lib.fnfreq (keep = firstname fn_uprob);
set lib.fnfreq;
attrib fn_uprob length = 8. format = 10.9;
fn_uprob = percent / 100;
run;
```

Calculate probabilistic weights

```
/* MATCH FIRST NAMES */

if firstname1 = firstname2 then fn_match = 'match';
else fn_match = 'nonmatch';

/* CALCULATE AGREEMENT WEIGHT FOR FIRST NAME AS:       */
/* LOG2(M_PROB/U_PROB)                                 */
/* ASSUME M-PROBABILITY FOR FIRST NAME = 0.95          */

if fn_match = 'match' then do;
  fn_agree_weight = log2(0.95 / fn_uprob);
end;

/* CALCULATE DISAGREEMENT WEIGHT FOR FIRST NAME AS:    */
/* LOG2( (1-M_PROB) / (1-U_PROB) )                     */
/* ASSUME M-PROBABILITY = 0.95                         */

else if fn_match = 'nonmatch' then do;
  fn_disagree_weight = log2( (1-0.95) / (1-fn_uprob) );
end;
```

Use editing distance method to calculate probability that two strings are a match

```
/* IF PROB. THAT 2 STRINGS ARE A MATCH > .95, THEN IT'S A MATCH */
if mean(
    1 - (length(firstname1) * spedis(firstname1, firstname2)) / 2400,
    1 - (length(firstname2) * spedis(firstname2, firstname1)) / 2400))
    >= .95
then firstname_spedis = 'match';
```
*** Source: "Fuzzy Key Linkage" by Sigurd Hermansen in Southeast SAS Users Group (2001) http://analytics.ncsu.edu/sesug/2001/P-816.pdf

Efficiency and Optimization Techniques

Syntax:
```
proc sql;
create index varname on datasetname (varname);
quit;
```

Ex. Create index on SSN to improve performance of match on SSN
```
proc sql;
create index ssn on dataset_a (ssn);
quit;

options msglevel = I;
proc sql;
create table matches as
select *
from dataset_a as f1, dataset_b as f2
where f1.ssn = f2.ssn;
quit;
```

Appendix 4.2. Data Linkage Software Packages

Manually writing the code to perform each step of the data linkage process in software packages such as SAS, MS SQL Server, or R gives the user full control over the entire process. While manual coding is ideal, the person writing the code must be familiar with linkage theory and must possess a great deal of programming expertise, qualities that may require funding for an expensive programmer. Furthermore, the amount of time required to write the code and the amount of computer resources needed to execute the linkage can be substantial. For researchers who lack the time, computer resources, expertise, or personnel required to write the needed code manually, many public-domain and commercial products are available to streamline and simplify the linkage process. Here, we present several commonly used products.

Publicly Available Packages

The following data linkage packages are available at no charge to the public:

Link Plus, developed by the Centers for Disease Control, is available at www.cdc.gov/cancer/npcr/tools/registryplus/lp.htm. The package provides a graphical user interface that is straightforward and easy to use, requiring only beginner-level knowledge of the linkage process. While Link Plus is easy to use, it may not be efficient or capable of processing large datasets (those with > 1 million records). This makes it difficult for researchers attempting to link claims datasets, which typically contain millions of records.

The Link King, developed by Washington State's Division of Alcohol and Substance Abuse, is available at www.the-link-king.com. The product itself is free, but it requires a license for base SAS, which currently costs ~ $2,000. Like Link Plus, the package provides a graphical user interface that is straightforward and easy to use, requiring only beginner-level knowledge of the linkage process.. While the Link King is capable of handling larger datasets, it requires first and last name, as well as Social Security Number or date of birth, which means that it can be used only in information-rich scenarios.

ChoiceMaker 2 (developed by ChoiceMaker Technologies and available at www.sourceforge.net/projects/oscmt/) and **FEBRL** (developed by the ANU Data Mining Group and available at www.sourceforge.net/projects/febrl/) are two products that health services researchers have used frequently in recent years. The authors are not aware of any scholarly evaluations of these products.

Commercially Available Products

Selected commercially available products are listed below:

LinkageWiz, developed by LinkageWiz Software, is available at www.linkagewiz.net/. The cost of LinkageWiz ranges from $199 for a 50,000 record limit to $2,999 for an unlimited record limit.

G-Link, developed by Statistics Canada, is available at http://www1.unece.org/stat/platform/display/msis/G-Link for $12,500 Canadian. This product is based on the probabilistic theory developed by William Winkler.

LinkSolv, developed by StrategicMatching, is available at www.strategicmatching.com/downloads.html.

Chapter 5. Evaluation of Methods Linking Health Registry Data to Insurance Claims in Scenarios of Varying Available Information

Objective

In this chapter, we expand upon our Chapter 4 discussion of linkage methods through an empirical linkage demonstration and evaluation using registry and insurance claims data. Here, we evaluate a set of linkage algorithms for registry-to-claims linkages covering scenarios of varying unique identifier availability and incorporate encryption algorithms to allow linkage without Protected Health Information transfer. We evaluated test algorithms against a gold standard used by the National Cancer Institute's Surveillance, Epidemiology and End Results (SEER)-Medicare program. More specifically, we examined linkage algorithms first with full identifying information including name and Social Security Number (SSN), then iterated through scenarios with decreasing numbers of unique identifiers and increasing reliance on nonunique information such as date of birth and sex. Given the exceptionally limited availability of practical empirical examples researchers can use to inform their own data linkages, this examination articulates much-needed specific details of the steps researchers may take and what they may expect to find given each study's unique scenario of data availability and quality.

Methods

Approach Overview

We compared four approaches:

1. Employment of the current *gold-standard* linking algorithm, first with full identifying information and subsequently with partial identifiers in place of their full counterparts

2a. Evaluation of *deterministic* approaches, modeling scenarios of decreasing individually identifiable information

2b. Evaluation of *deterministic* approaches in the context of *encrypted* individual identifiers, simulating a scenario of restrictions on identifier release to researchers

3. Evaluation of *probabilistic* approaches, modeling scenarios of decreasing individually identifiable information

Experimental linkage sets start with full available information and iteratively reduce the available information, in the end simulating a scenario in which unique identifiers are not available. To both streamline this examination and test the robustness of the algorithms in the context of the rareness of the condition of interest, we begin by focusing on a sample (subpopulation) with colon cancer, a common sex-neutral cancer. Next, we examine cancers that are rarer and sex specific. Finally, we evaluate algorithm performance in the context of all cancers simultaneously in the full health-plan claims population. Table 5.1 provides an overview of our approach.

Table 5.1. Overview of experimental linkage approach

Approach	Maximum Available Information and Unique Individual Identifiers (Gold Standard)	→→→		Incrementally Reduced Information, No Unique Individual Identifiers (Experimental Sets)
1. Deterministic linkage	Linkage 1.1	Linkage 1.2	.. ..	Linkage 1.n
2. Deterministic with encryption	Linkage 2.1	Linkage 2.2	.. ..	Linkage 2.n
3. Probabilistic linkage	Linkage 3.1	Linkage 3.2	.. ..	Linkage 3.n

Data Sources and Patient Populations

Case data: Individuals in the North Carolina Central Cancer Registry (NCCCR) diagnosed with colon cancer in the period 2007–08 (n = 6,444 unique individuals)

Claims data: Enrollment and claims data for beneficiaries in privately insured health plans in North Carolina (PAYER) for the period 2006–09 (n = 3,747,250 unique beneficiaries)

We selected these datasets because they have full information (i.e., all identifying variables) commonly captured in constituent datasets for linkages of this nature. The variables in the claims data are the same as those available in the Federal payer/claims data. Registry records were matched to all years of PAYER claims. The PAYER claims data can be restricted to simulate practical scenarios of comparatively limited linking information experienced by researchers.

Table 5.2 shows identifiers available in both datasets.

Table 5.2. Variables available for linkage and their completeness in study datasets

Variable	Alternative Forms	Completeness	
		NCCCR (%)	PAYER (%)
SSN	SSN4; SSN2	99.7	89.3
Last name	Last name initial (LNI); Last name Soundex (LNS)	100.0	100.0
First name	First name initial (FNI); first name Soundex (FNS)	100.0	99.9
Date of birth	Month and year of birth; year of birth; DOB2	100.0	100.0
Sex		100.0	100.0
Residence	County of residence; ZIP Code of residence	99.9	99.9
Diagnosis	Valid diagnosis code Diagnosis category (e.g., any cancer) Specific diagnosis (e.g., colon cancer)	100.0	100.0 28.1 2.9

DOB2 = any 2 of 3 date of birth parts match; NCCCR = North Carolina Central Cancer Registry; PAYER = data for beneficiaries in privately insured health plans in North Carolina; SSN = Social Security Number; SSN2 = last 2 digits of SSN; SSN4 = last 4 digits of SSN.

Chapter 5. Evaluation of Methods Linking Health Registry Data to Insurance Claims in Scenarios of Varying Available Information

Data Cleaning and Standardization

Before the linkage, variables were cleaned and standardized as follows:

1. All string variables were converted to uppercase and stripped of all punctuation and digits, and hyphenated names were broken out into two different name fields.
2. All date variables were converted to date9. format (e.g., 01SEP2013).
3. ZIP Codes were limited to the first 5 digits.
4. FIPS (Federal Information Processing Standards) codes were broken out into State (first 2 digits) and county (last 3 digits) codes.
5. Invalid SSNs were flagged and treated as missing.

Data Linkage

Blocking Phase. Rather than consider the Cartesian product of all possible matches between NCCCR and PAYER, we identified a subset of potential matches during an initial blocking phase. Two records were included in the subset of potential matches if they agreed on any of the following:

1. SSN
2. Date of birth, first name initial, and sex
3. Date of birth, last name initial, and sex
4. Last name, first name, and sex
5. Date of birth, county, and sex

The blocking phase identified 104,360 possible matches.

Step 1. Application of a Gold-Standard Algorithm. At this time, because there is presently no definitive gold-standard algorithm for registry linkages, we used the linkage algorithm developed by the National Cancer Institute's SEER-Medicare program as a gold standard.[82] The iterative deterministic approach employed in this algorithm has demonstrated high validity and reliability in previous registry-to-claims linkages, has been employed successfully in numerous updates of the SEER-Medicare linked dataset, and is generally perceived to be strong in scenarios of high data quality and identifier completeness.[80-82]

Individuals in the NCCCR database were linked to beneficiaries in the PAYER database using the SEER-Medicare algorithm, which consists of a sequence of deterministic matches using different match criteria in each successive round:

In the first step, records were declared a match if they agreed on SSN and one of the following:

- First and last name (allowing for fuzzy matches, such as nicknames);
- Last name, month of birth, and sex; or
- First name, month of birth, and sex.

If SSN was missing or did not match, or two records failed to meet the initial match criteria, they were subjected to a second round of deterministic linkages. In the second round, records were declared a match if they agreed on last name, first name, month of birth, sex, and one of the following:

- 7-9 digits of the SSN; or
- Two or more of: year of birth, day of birth, middle initial, or date of death.

For each pair of records, match or nonmatch status was determined using the rules above, and match markers were generated indicating agreement or disagreement on each individual identifier. The SEER-Medicare algorithm classified 1,189 record pairs as matches and 103,171 record pairs as nonmatches. Based on prior knowledge of cancer incidence and insurance coverage in North Carolina, we expected that approximately 20 percent of individuals in the NCCCR database with colon cancer would be insured by PAYER. The 1,189 uniquely matched individuals represent 18.5 percent of the individuals with colon cancer identified in the NCCCR database.

All subsequent test algorithms were evaluated against the SEER-Medicare algorithm. The match decisions made by each algorithm were compared with the match decisions made through use of the gold-standard algorithm. Pairs identified as matches by both the SEER-Medicare algorithm and the test algorithm were declared to be "true matches." Pairs identified as matches by the SEER-Medicare algorithm and nonmatches by the test algorithm were declared to be "false nonmatches." Pairs identified as nonmatches by both the SEER-Medicare algorithm and the test algorithm were declared to be "true nonmatches." Pairs identified as nonmatches by the SEER-Medicare algorithm and matches by the test algorithm were declared to be "false matches."

To assess the success of each algorithm, we calculated sensitivity, positive predictive value, and f-measure (where beta was set at 1.0, giving equal weight to sensitivity and specificity) using SAS (version 9.3; SAS Institute, Cary, NC).

Step 2a. Comparison Approach 1—Deterministic Linking. Deterministic linkage strategies have been recommended for situations in which the data are of high quality and/or many identifier variables are available.[59] Research has also shown that deterministic linkage on a sufficient number of partial and/or indirect identifiers, such as initials, year of birth, and county of residence, can provide sufficient discriminatory power to classify matches and nonmatches with good sensitivity and specificity.[42,72]

Using the matching markers generated above, we developed and tested a set of deterministic algorithms, using match variable combinations of full and partial identifiers. We covered information-rich situations in which full direct identifiers (e.g., SSNs and full names) are available, as well as information-poor situations in which only indirect or partial identifiers are available. Only record pairs that were uniquely identified by the given variable combination were considered potential matches. When multiple record pairs matched on the values of a given variable combination, the record pairs were flagged as ties and classified as nonmatches. To account for minor typographical errors in names, we used the Soundex algorithm to generate a code consisting of the first initial and up to three digits representing consonant sounds in the name, and matched on the Soundex values. By doing so, we were able to explore the possibility of linking algorithms that do not require the release of full or actual names.

Following Roos and Wajda, we determined the percentage of records identified uniquely by each combination of variables.[63] Given the exploratory nature of this study, we relaxed the recommended threshold of ~1.00 record per unique value (100% uniqueness) and included for testing all variable combinations that identified 85 percent of records uniquely. Using this method, we selected 398 variable combinations for testing. To simulate scenarios of decreasing information availability, the variables with the largest number of unique values were removed in a stepwise manner. The first group of algorithms used all identifiers. The second group of algorithms excluded SSN. Finally, the third group of identifiers excluded SSN and name.

Step 2b. Comparison Approach 1—Encryption Variation. In situations where full identifiers or partial identifiers are available but may not be released or transmitted, research has shown that records can be successfully linked via deterministic algorithms using identifiers encrypted before release.[45,47,85,86] To simulate the application of a hash encryption method before release, we converted the variable combinations presented in Step 2a to 128-bit hash values using the md5 algorithm. Each conversion was performed using the md5 function in SAS 9.3. It is important to note that the length, format, order, and content of the strings in the two datasets have to be perfectly consistent before the conversion. If there is even a slight difference between the two strings, the md5 algorithm will generate two different values, as shown in Table 5.3 below.

Chapter 5. Evaluation of Methods Linking Health Registry Data to Insurance Claims in Scenarios of Varying Available Information

Table 5.3. Example md5 algorithm values from inconsistent strings

Source	Date of Birth	First Name	Last Name	MD5 Code
NCCCR	12312013	BILL	SMITH	<DgiÖ oÓĺi=$2e'Ä
PAYER	12312013	Bill	Smith	*Ym1" Ö¼åëÑðÁ@

NCCCR = North Carolina Central Cancer Registry; PAYER = data for beneficiaries in privately insured health plans in North Carolina.

While the two records in this example clearly match on date of birth, first name, and last name, the md5 hash values for the two concatenated strings are very different due to the different casing on the names. Both strings would need to be ordered, formatted, and spaced uniformly for the md5 algorithm to generate the same value for the two strings. Using the example above, the best approach would be to standardize nicknames, concatenate the three identifiers, remove all spaces, and convert the case of the names to uppercase (i.e., '12312013BILLSMITH') before applying the md5 algorithm. We performed a deterministic match on the hash values for each variable combination presented in Step 2a.

Step 3. Comparison Approach 2—Probabilistic Linking. Probabilistic linkage strategies have been recommended for situations in which the data contain many coding errors and/or only a few identifiers are available.[63] Using the match markers generated earlier, we developed and tested a set of probabilistic algorithms using the match variable combinations in each group of full and partial identifiers that performed best in Step 2a. We covered information-rich situations in which full direct identifiers (e.g., SSNs and full names) are available, as well as information-poor situations in which only indirect or partial identifiers are available. Only record pairs that were uniquely identified by the given variable combination were considered potential matches. When multiple record pairs matched on the values of a given variable combination, the record pairs were flagged as ties and classified as nonmatches. The goal in this step is to improve on the match results in Step 2a by making use of the information ignored in deterministic algorithms. A summary of steps for probabilistic record linkage is provided in Chapter 4.

For each matched pair, we calculated agreement weights and disagreement weights for each identifier. Following the Fellegi and Sunter model,[33] agreement weights were calculated by dividing the probability that true matches agree on the specific value of the identifier by the probability that false matches randomly agree on the specific value of the identifier, and taking the $\log_2$ of the quotient. For example, if the probability that true matches agree on month of birth is 97 percent and the probability that false matches randomly agree on month of birth is 8.3 percent (1/12), then the agreement weight for month of birth would be $\log_2(.97/.083)$, or 3.54. Disagreement weights were calculated by dividing 1 minus the probability that true matches agree on the specific value of the identifier by 1 minus the probability that false matches agree on the specific value of the identifier, and taking the $\log_2$ of the quotient.

To allow for comparisons across linkage strategies, we tested the same 398 variable combinations that were selected for testing in Step 2a. The linkage score for each matched pair was then computed as the sum of the weights. Using the method developed by Cook et al.,[44] we calculated the threshold weight needed to achieve a 95-percent probability that two matched records are a true match. Matched pairs with a linkage score greater than the threshold weight were declared "matches," while matched pairs with a linkage score less than the threshold weight were declared "nonmatches." We present results from the top five algorithms.

Results

Gold-Standard Linkage

The SEER-Medicare algorithm, using full identifiers, classified 1,189 record pairs as matches and 103,171 record pairs as nonmatches. In a stepwise fashion, we replaced the full identifiers with partial identifiers to determine whether the algorithm can work in the absence of full identifiers. Selected results of the SEER-Medicare iterative deterministic algorithm with full identifiers replaced with the indicated partial identifiers are presented in Table 5.4. The results indicate that the sensitivity of the algorithm was largely unaffected in the five examples presented in the table. The replacement of full identifiers with partial identifiers, however, did slightly increase the number of false matches. (Note that manual review confirmed that the additional matches identified by the algorithms with partial identifiers were in fact nonmatches.) Despite the small decrease in the specificity of the algorithm (not shown), these results indicate that the SEER-Medicare linkage can perform effectively in the absence of full identifiers.

Table 5.4. Selected results of gold-standard linkage algorithm with partial identifiers

Linking Variables	Matches		Nonmatches		Sensitivity	PPV	F-Measure
	True	False	True	False			
Algorithm 1	1,186	14	103,157	3	99.75	98.83	99.29
Algorithm 2	1,185	13	103,158	4	99.66	98.91	99.28
Algorithm 3	1,189	19	103,152	0	100.00	98.43	99.21
Algorithm 4	1,171	9	103,162	18	98.49	99.24	98.86
Algorithm 5	1,171	14	103,157	18	98.49	98.82	98.65

PPV = positive predictive value.

Descriptions of the gold-standard algorithms follow.

Algorithm 1: Criteria for classifying a match–

Individuals match on last 4 of SSN <u>and</u> one of the following sets of criteria:

1. First name Soundex, last name Soundex, 2 out of 3 DOB (date of birth) parts
2. Last name Soundex, 2 out of 3 DOB parts, sex
3. First name Soundex, 2 out of 3 DOB parts, sex

OR

Individuals <u>do not</u> match on last 4 digits of SSN, but match on last name Soundex, first name Soundex, 2 out of 3 DOB parts, sex, <u>and</u> one of the following sets of criteria:

1. Middle initial or date of death
2. ZIP Code or county
3. Primary cancer site

Algorithm 2: Criteria for classifying a match–

Individuals match on last 4 of SSN <u>and</u> one of the following sets of criteria:

1. First name Soundex, last name Soundex, 2 out of 3 DOB parts
2. Last name Soundex, 2 out of 3 DOB parts, sex
3. First name Soundex, 2 out of 3 DOB parts, sex

OR

Individuals <u>do not</u> match on last 4 digits of SSN, but match on last name Soundex, first name

Soundex, 2 out of 3 DOB parts, sex, <u>and</u> one of the following sets of criteria:

1. Middle initial or date of death
2. County

Algorithm 3: Criteria for classifying a match–

Individuals match on last 4 of SSN <u>and</u> one of the following sets of criteria:

1. First name Soundex, last name Soundex
2. Last name Soundex, 2 out of 3 DOB parts, sex
3. First name Soundex, 2 out of 3 DOB parts, sex

OR

Individuals <u>do not</u> match on last 4 digits of SSN, but match on last name Soundex, first name Soundex, month of birth, sex, <u>and</u> one of the following sets of criteria:

- Two of the following match: year of birth, day of birth, middle initial, or date of death

Algorithm 4: Criteria for classifying a match–

Individuals match on last 4 of SSN <u>and</u> one of the following sets of criteria:

1. First name Soundex, last name Soundex, 2 out of 3 DOB parts
2. Last name Soundex, 2 out of 3 DOB parts, sex
3. First name Soundex, 2 out of 3 DOB parts, sex

OR

Individuals <u>do not</u> match on last 4 digits of SSN, but match on one of the following sets of criteria:

1. Last name Soundex, first name Soundex, DOB, sex
2. Last name Soundex, 2 of 3 DOB parts, ZIP Code, sex, (middle initial or date of death)
3. First name Soundex, 2 of 3 DOB parts, ZIP Code, sex, (middle initial or date of death)

Algorithm 5: Criteria for classifying a match–

Individuals match on last 4 digits of SSN <u>and</u> one of the following sets of criteria:

1. First name Soundex, last name Soundex, 2 out of 3 DOB parts
2. Last name Soundex, 2 out of 3 DOB parts, sex
3. First name Soundex, 2 out of 3 DOB parts, sex

OR

Individuals <u>do not</u> match on last 4 digits of SSN, but match on one of the following sets of criteria:

1. Last name Soundex, first name Soundex, DOB, sex
2. Last name Soundex, 2 of 3 DOB parts, ZIP Code, sex

Deterministic Linkage

Results of the deterministic linkages are presented in Table 5.5. The relatively lower sensitivity scores (87.13–88.39) for algorithms using SSN reflect the fact that only 89 percent of the private payer's members had a valid SSN listed. As expected, algorithms using SSN have very high specificity (99.99–100.00) and positive predictive value (99.33–99.90).

When we excluded SSN, the best performing algorithms were able to identify correctly more matches (85.70–92.26) without sacrificing specificity (99.99–100.00), and with only minor decreases in positive predictive value (99.03–100.00). The most encouraging result is the finding that DOB, last name Soundex, first name Soundex, and sex correctly and uniquely identified 92 percent of matches identified by the SEER-Medicare algorithm, with specificity and positive predictive value over 99 percent. Preferably, all values would be greater than 95 percent, but this finding demonstrates that a good linkage can be performed in the absence of SSN or actual name. Importantly, exclusion of a linkage variable may reduce the number of matches in some cases if it results in a greater number of ties. This is demonstrated in Table 5.5 when comparing algorithms without unique identifiers such as SSN, name, and DOB, where inclusion of the variable "sex" resulted in 552 true matches and exclusion resulted in only 541 matches.

The sensitivity of algorithms that did not include SSN or name was significantly lower than that of algorithms that did include SSN and/or name. However, algorithms that blocked on primary site (e.g., diagnosis code for colon cancer) demonstrated high specificity (99.96–99.99) and high positive predictive value (95.09–99.59) (data not shown).

Results of the deterministic linkage approaches using encryption are presented in Table 5.6. The results for each algorithm were consistent with the previous results (Table 5.5), indicating that a deterministic match on identifiers encrypted before release can be successful in instances where identifiers are available but not releasable.

Table 5.5. Selected results of deterministic linkage algorithms

Linking Variables	Matches		Nonmatches		Sensitivity	PPV	F-Measure
	True	False	True	False			
Combinations That Include SSN							
SSN4 and month of birth	1,051	6	103,165	138	88.39	99.43	93.59
SSN4 and year of birth	1,048	4	103,167	141	88.14	99.62	93.53
SSN and month of birth	1,041	3	103,168	148	87.55	99.71	93.24
SSN and sex	1,043	7	103,164	146	87.72	99.33	93.16
SSN and year of birth	1,036	1	103,170	153	87.13	99.90	93.08
Combinations Excluding SSN							
DOB, FNS, LNS, and sex	1,097	5	103,166	92	92.26	99.55	95.77
DOB, FN, LN, and sex	1,087	0	103,171	102	91.42	100.00	95.52
DOB2, FNS, LNS, county, and sex	1,029	9	103,168	160	86.54	99.13	92.41
DOB, LN, county, and sex	1,020	5	103,166	169	86.12	99.51	92.33
DOB, LNS, county, and sex	1,019	10	103,161	170	85.70	99.03	91.88
Combinations Excluding SSN and Name							
DX, DOB2, ZIP, and sex	839	12	103,159	350	70.56	99.59	82.60
DX, DOB, county, and sex	841	29	103,142	348	70.73	96.67	81.69
DX, DOB, ZIP, and sex	824	9	103,162	365	69.30	98.92	81.50
DX, year of birth, ZIP, and sex	813	9	103,162	376	68.38	98.19	80.62
DX, month of birth, ZIP, and sex	749	8	103,163	440	62.99	98.94	76.97
Combinations Excluding SSN, Name, and DOB							
DX, ZIP, MI, and sex	552	3	103,168	637	46.43	99.46	63.31
DX, ZIP, and MI	541	3	103,168	648	45.50	99.45	62.43
DX, county, MI, and sex	394	4	103,167	795	33.14	98.99	49.66
DX, county, and MI	333	3	103,168	856	28.01	99.11	43.68
DX, ZIP, and sex	332	4	103,167	857	27.92	98.91	43.55

DOB = date of birth; DOB2 = 2 of 3 DOB parts; DX = diagnosis; FN = first name; FNS = first name Soundex; LN = last name; LNS = last name Soundex; MI = middle initial; PPV = positive predictive value; SSN = Social Security Number; SSN4 = last 4 digits of SSN.

Chapter 5. Evaluation of Methods Linking Health Registry Data to Insurance Claims in Scenarios of Varying Available Information

Probabilistic Linkage

As shown in Table 5.7, the probabilistic approach improved the performance of all algorithms. When all identifiers were included, the sensitivity improved from ~87 percent to 97.92 percent, because many of the ~13 percent of the private payer's members' missing SSNs were matched using information provided by matches on other identifiers.

This demonstrates the ability of probabilistic algorithms to perform well when data quality for some identifiers is poor. In this instance, missing information in one important identifier was overcome by information provided in other identifiers, thus improving the sensitivity and accuracy of the probabilistic approach compared with a deterministic approach. While the iterative deterministic approach used in the SEER-Medicare algorithm is similarly able to overcome poor data quality in an important identifier such as SSN, it relies on SSN and full name. Conversely, probabilistic algorithms can be effective in scenarios where SSN and full name are unavailable, as demonstrated by the second probabilistic algorithm reported in Table 5.5. Using only DOB, first and last name Soundex values, residence, diagnosis, and sex, the probabilistic approach was able to identify correctly 96.67 percent of true matches and 99.99 percent of true nonmatches. Thus, if confidentiality concerns block the release of SSN and full name in the future, registry data can still be linked successfully to claims using the probabilistic approach. The final results reported in Table 5.7 show that algorithms relying solely on DOB, residence, diagnosis, and sex were unsuccessful, although the probabilistic approach showed some improvement over the deterministic approach. Additional information not used in this study (e.g., service dates) may provide a probabilistic approach with the added power needed for a successful linkage without SSN or name Soundex values.

Table 5.6. Selected results of deterministic linkage algorithms using encrypted data

	Matches		Nonmatches				
Linking Variables	True	False	True	False	Sensitivity	PPV	F-Measure
Combinations That Include SSN							
SSN4 and month of birth	1,051	6	103,165	138	88.39	99.43	93.59
SSN4 and year of birth	1,048	4	103,167	141	88.14	99.62	93.53
SSN and month of birth	1,041	3	103,168	148	87.55	99.71	93.24
SSN and sex	1,043	7	103,164	146	87.72	99.33	93.16
SSN and year of birth	1,036	1	103,170	153	87.13	99.90	93.08
Combinations Excluding SSN							
DOB, FNS, LNS, and sex	1,097	5	103,166	92	92.26	99.55	95.77
DOB, FN, LN, and sex	1,087	0	103,171	102	91.42	100.00	95.52
DOB2, FNS, LNS, county, and sex	1,029	9	103,168	160	86.54	99.13	92.41
DOB, LN, county, and sex	1,020	5	103,166	169	86.12	99.51	92.33
DOB, LNS, county, and sex	1,019	10	103,161	170	85.70	99.03	91.88
Combinations Excluding SSN and Name							
DX, DOB2, ZIP, and sex	839	12	103,159	350	70.56	99.59	82.60
DX, DOB, county, and sex	841	29	103,142	348	70.73	96.67	81.69
DX, DOB, ZIP, and sex	824	9	103,162	365	69.30	98.92	81.50
DX, year of birth, ZIP, and sex	813	9	103,162	376	68.38	98.19	80.62
DX, month of birth, ZIP, and sex	749	8	103,163	440	62.99	98.94	76.97
Combinations Excluding SSN, Name, and DOB							
DX, ZIP, MI, and sex	552	3	103,168	637	46.43	99.46	63.31
DX, ZIP, and MI	541	3	103,168	648	45.50	99.45	62.43
DX, county, MI, and sex	394	4	103,167	795	33.14	98.99	49.66
DX, county, and MI	333	3	103,168	856	28.01	99.11	43.68
DX, ZIP, and sex	332	4	103,167	857	27.92	98.91	43.55

DOB = date of birth; DOB2 = 2 of 3 DOB parts; DX = diagnosis; FN = first name; FNS = first name Soundex; LN = last name; LNS = last name Soundex; MI = middle initial; PPV = positive predictive value; SSN = Social Security Number; SSN4 = last 4 digits of SSN.

Table 5.7. Selected results of probabilistic linkage algorithms

Linking Variables	Matches		Nonmatches		Sensitivity	PPV	F-Measure
	True	False	True	False			
Combinations That Include SSN							
SSN4, FN, LN, DOB, county, and sex	1,171	7	103,164	18	98.49	99.41	98.95
SSN4, FN, LN, DOB, ZIP, and sex	1,171	8	103,163	18	98.48	99.32	98.90
SSN, FN, LN, DOB, ZIP, and sex	1,171	8	103,163	18	98.48	99.32	98.90
SSN, FNS, LNS, DOB, ZIP, and sex	1,169	8	103,163	20	98.32	99.32	98.82
SSN4, FNS, LNS, DOB, ZIP, and sex	1,168	8	103,163	21	98.23	99.32	98.77
Combinations Excluding SSN							
DOB, LN, FN, ZIP, and sex	1,147	10	103,161	42	96.47	99.14	97.79
DOB, LN, FN, county, and sex	1,136	9	103,162	53	95.54	99.21	97.34
DOB, LNS, FNS, county, and sex	1,119	9	103,162	70	94.11	99.93	96.93
DOB, LNS, FNS, ZIP, and sex	1,131	14	103,157	58	95.12	98.78	96.92
DOB, LN, ZIP, and sex	1,033	10	103,161	156	86.88	99.04	92.56
Combinations Excluding SSN and Name							
DX, DOB, ZIP, MI, and sex	885	22	103,149	304	74.43	97.57	84.44
DX, DOB2, ZIP, MI, and sex	865	17	103,154	324	72.75	98.07	83.53
DX, DOB, ZIP, and sex	830	9	103,162	359	69.81	98.93	81.86
DX, DOB, county, and sex	844	29	103,142	345	70.98	96.68	81.86
DX, year of birth, ZIP, and sex	818	9	103,162	371	68.71	98.91	81.09
Combinations Excluding SSN, Name, and DOB							
DX, ZIP, MI, and sex	765	10	103,161	424	64.34	98.71	77.90
DX, ZIP, and MI	719	7	103,164	470	60.47	99.04	75.09
DX, county, MI, and sex	634	9	103,162	555	53.12	98.60	69.04
DX, county, and MI	333	3	103,168	856	28.01	99.11	43.68
DX, ZIP, and sex	333	4	103,167	856	28.01	98.81	43.65

DOB = date of birth; DOB2 = 2 of 3 DOB parts; DX = diagnosis; FN = first name; FNS = first name Soundex; LN = last name; LNS = last name Soundex; MI = middle initial; PPV = positive predictive value; SSN = Social Security Number; SSN4 = last 4 digits of SSN.

Discussion

The results of this study indicate that a successful linkage is possible in the absence of full identifying information. We found that straightforward and easy-to-employ deterministic algorithms using DOB and Soundex codes for names demonstrated high specificity and positive predictive value with acceptable sensitivity. In situations where identifiers are available, but not allowed to be released, we found that deterministic matching on hash-encrypted variable combinations performed as well as deterministic matching on the same combination of unencrypted variables. However, the performance of the hash-encrypted deterministic match requires that the variables within each dataset be cleaned and standardized in exactly the same way, and the exact linkage method needs to be known ahead of time. Thus, data-providing organizations have to commit more effort and coordination to collaboratively determine the best standardization methods and combination of variables to use for the linkage before the encryption can be carried out in each of the organizations.

In information-rich scenarios where identifiers are available for release, iterative deterministic approaches such as the SEER-Medicare algorithm are highly effective, and much more time and resource efficient than probabilistic approaches, which can be highly complex and difficult to implement. However, when unique identifiers such as SSN and full name are unavailable, the probabilistic approach consistently outperforms the deterministic approach. These findings are particularly important, as confidentiality concerns are making it increasingly difficult to obtain identifying information for linkage projects.

Appendix 5.1. SEER-Medicare Algorithm With Partial Identifiers

Abbreviations: DOB = date of birth; SEER = Surveillance, Epidemiology and End Results; SSN = Social Security Number.

Algorithm 1:

If last 4 digits of SSN match, then
    if first name Soundex, last name Soundex, 2 out of 3 DOB parts match
    or
    if last name Soundex, 2 out of 3 DOB parts, sex match
    or
    if first name Soundex, 2 out of 3 DOB parts, sex match,
        then it's a match.

If last 4 digits of SSN do not match, then
    if last name Soundex, first name Soundex, 2 out of 3 DOB parts, sex match, then
        if sum(of middle initial, date of death) >= 1
        or
        if sum(of ZIP, county) >= 1
        or
        if primary_site match,
then it's a match.

Algorithm 2:

If last 4 digits of SSN match, then
    if first name Soundex, last name Soundex, 2 out of 3 DOB parts match
    or
    if last name Soundex, 2 out of 3 DOB parts, sex match
    or
    if first name Soundex, 2 out of 3 DOB parts, sex match,
    then it's a match.

If last 4 digits of SSN do not match, then
    if last name Soundex, first name Soundex, 2 out of 3 DOB parts, sex match, then
    if sum(of middle initial, date of death) >= 1
    or
    county,
    then it's a match.

Algorithm 3:

If last 4 digits of SSN match, then
    if first name Soundex, last name Soundex match
    or
    last name Soundex, 2 of 3 DOB parts, sex match
    or
    first name Soundex, 2 out of 3 DOB parts, sex match,
    then it's a match.

If last 4 digits of SSN do not match, then
    if last name Soundex, first name Soundex, month of birth, sex match
    or
    if (sum(of year of birth, day of birth, middle initial, date of death) >= 2),
    then it's a match.

Algorithm 4:

If last 4 digits of SSN match, then
    if first name Soundex, last name Soundex, 2 out of 3 DOB parts match
    or
    if last name Soundex, 2 out of 3 DOB parts, sex match
    or
    if first name Soundex, 2 out of 3 DOB parts, sex match,
    then it's a match.

Linking Data for Health Services Research

If last 4 digits of SSN do not match, then
    if last name Soundex, first name Soundex, DOB, sex match
    or
    if last name Soundex, 2 out 3 DOB parts, ZIP, sex, (middle initial or date of death) match
    or
    if first name Soundex, 2 out 3 DOB parts, ZIP, sex, (middle initial or date of death) match;
    then it's a match.

Algorithm 5:

If last 4 digits of SSN match, then
    if first name Soundex, last name Soundex, 2 out of 3 DOB parts match
    or
    if last name Soundex, 2 out of 3 DOB parts, sex match
    or
    if first name Soundex, 2 out of 3 DOB parts, sex match,
    then it's a match.

If last 4 digits of SSN do not match, then
    if last name Soundex, first name Soundex, DOB, sex match
    or
    if last name Soundex, 2 out 3 DOB parts, ZIP, sex match,
    then it's a match.

Chapter 6. Project Summary and Recommendations for Researchers

Overview

Randomized controlled trials (RCTs) remain the gold standard for assessing intervention efficacy; however, RCT results often cannot be generalized due to a lack of inclusion of "real-world" combinations of interventions and heterogeneous patients.[1-4] With recent advances in information technology, data, and statistical methods, there is tremendous promise in leveraging ever-growing repositories of secondary data to support comparative effectiveness and public health research. While there are many advantages to using these secondary data sources, they are often limited in scope, which in turn limits their utility in addressing important questions in a comprehensive manner. These limitations can be overcome by linking data from multiple sources such as health registries and administrative claims data.[6,7,9]

This report provides a conceptual framework for high-quality data linkage in the context of comparative effectiveness research (CER). It describes the infrastructure and personnel needed to navigate the linkage process, outlines the Data Use Agreement process, presents different approaches to data linkage, discusses the strengths and weaknesses of each, and makes recommendations on which approaches perform best in varying scenarios of data availability. In this report, researchers have a step-by-step instructional guide for designing new CER studies that involve linking patient registries with other secondary data sources. We also highlight considerations for researchers, data managers, information technology managers, and other stakeholders likely to be involved in the data linkage process.

Considerations for Project Planning

Appropriateness and Feasibility of the Project

Each data source needs to be considered carefully regarding its adequacy for the specific linkage endeavor. First and foremost, the *quality* and *discriminatory power* of each of the available linkage identifiers need to be scrutinized. Second, researchers must be confident that there is enough overlap in the two populations to merit the effort. Every linkage will result in a set of matches that will serve as a select, nonrandom, and perhaps not completely representative sample of the two disparate underlying populations. It is important that the extent and representativeness of this potential overlap be considered before beginning the process. Finally, it must be evident that the linkage will result in an enriched dataset that includes additional data elements made possible only through the linkage. Each of these considerations must be weighed together as a whole to determine whether the linkage will provide an adequate return on the investment in time and resources.

Data Ownership and Governance

Before proposing a linkage, it must be clear that each of the respective data sources allows for the scope of the proposed work. All data owners or key stakeholders need to be contacted, and existing data-governance processes need to be understood. Rules regarding consent and any existing regulatory requirements for the data need to be clarified. The importance of these issues should not be underestimated, and the logistical, administrative, and often legal hurdles need to be anticipated and built into the cost and the timeline for the project.

Technical Environment and Security

A secure and well-performing computing platform represents the operational backbone for conducting innovative research using large datasets. There is a fine balance between security and usability, and system performance directly influences the size and complexity of the data that can be managed and linked. Careful planning and building collaborations with teams with technical resources help decrease the cost/benefit ratio, while allowing growth in the future. As outlined in Chapter 2, a well-performing and secure research environment builds a foundation of trust with research partners and data suppliers.

Team, Skills, and Expertise

The complexity and scope of a research project will dictate the type of team and expertise required. As scope and complexity increase, the required experience and expertise of team members narrow and deepen. Ideally, a research and data support team will already be in place before the proposal process. These individuals can provide essential insight into considerations such as feasibility, technical environment, approach, and linkage processes, all of which are identified in this report. Specific and key roles have been outlined in Chapter 2. For nearly all data linkage projects, the research team should include individuals with experience developing and evaluating linking algorithms, as well as overall expertise in population research. Other technical skills are no less essential for project success. For example, a knowledgeable data manager will be able to evaluate the appropriateness of the datasets, assess the computational feasibility of the linkage, estimate computing requirements, and develop a common data model. Information or computing technology experts can help design, run, and optimize the required technical environment and computing platform. Lastly, any large linkage project will require a conscientious and knowledgeable project manager who is experienced in the many security standards and legal documents and processes that are required to get the project off the ground and keep it moving throughout its life course.

Cost

Several financial considerations need to be incorporated into project planning and execution for any linkage project. First, obtaining a copy of the data or purchasing a user license often comes with a hefty price. Second, the information technology (IT) systems and technical platform requirements are often significant and can be expensive to build and maintain. However, other options may be available besides building a system de novo. Renting infrastructure from another research partner or computing environment, or utilizing a third-party vendor for data linkage, may provide cost savings and synergy at an organizational level. Lastly, the technical personnel required for linking and maintaining data are often in high demand in this era of "big data" and may require high salaries for recruitment and retention.

Identification and Evaluation of Available Linkage Keys

The quantity, quality, and discriminatory power of available identifiers will determine the feasibility and success of any linking endeavor. This information may or may not be known before data delivery but can often be estimated. Chapter 3 outlines different types of identifiers and key aspects of each, and identifies factors to consider when weighing the feasibility of a proposed linkage project. The quality, completeness, and predictive ability of each of the potential keys must be assessed separately in each respective dataset, with careful attention paid to missing, invalid, or implausible values. This effort will drive the choice of the appropriate data linkage strategy.

Chapter 6. Project Summary and Recommendations for Researchers

Variable Cleaning, Standardization, and a Common Data Model (Normalization)

To begin cleaning and standardizing variables before linking, it is vital that the researchers obtain and review all available reference documentation (e.g., literature search, gray literature) so the research team understands the underlying intent and purpose of the data as well as the origination of the variables. These aspects of the original data directly affect the quality of the variables and drive later decisions about the appropriate linkage method. The amount of data cleaning and standardization needed depends on the quality and source of the data as well as the researcher's question and available resources. Chapter 4 of this report outlines some of the common standardization measures required to prepare the linkage identifiers. Each key variable comes with its own idiosyncrasies, and thus a specific standardization and cleaning protocol must be developed and documented for each key. For example, decisions regarding standardization of format (e.g., dates set to "mmddyyyy"), case (e.g.., all uppercase), punctuation (e.g., remove dashes from Social Security Number [SSN]), and missing values (e.g., use a consistent value such as quotation marks ['] or periods [.] or other common values to denote missing [9999]) need to be made and documented. In some cases, secondary software or datasets (crosswalk files) may help to standardize or clean the variables (e.g., through linkage to common nicknames or synonyms).

Downstream from standardizing and cleaning identifiers, but important in preparing the data for linkage, is the development of a common data model. As the data are prepared for linkage and subsequent use, researchers need to understand, outline, define, and document the division of the data into separate subtables, as well as the relationships between tables within the linked dataset (i.e., entity relationships). This involves the development of a procedure for joining tables (e.g., assignment of a primary key) and determining whether the relationships of the individuals within these tables are one to one, one to many, many to one, or many to many. Finally, decisions regarding variables that are repeated across datasets need to be made. Elements such as sex, race, and dates are often stored in different formats and need to be standardized in the linked dataset. Furthermore, protocols for handling discrepancies (e.g., different birth dates or race categories) across data sources need to be developed and documented.

Linkage Approach

Once the researchers have familiarized themselves with the relevant data sources and evaluated the available linkage variables, they can make an initial determination about the most appropriate data linkage strategy. Chapters 4 and 5 outline different linkage approaches and discuss the strengths and weaknesses of each approach. The first step in selecting the appropriate linkage strategy is to determine whether direct unique identifiers are available (e.g., SSNs). In scenarios in which direct unique identifiers are available, deemed to be of high quality, and nonmissing in approximately 95 percent of cases in each dataset, a deterministic approach is recommended. A one-time deterministic approach is the easiest to design, implement, and interpret. It involves a binary, "all or nothing" decisionmaking process in which record pairs are compared character for character across all identifiers. Record pairs that agree exactly on the given identifiers are classified as matches, while record pairs that disagree on even a single character are classified as nonmatches. This approach does not account for the differential *discriminatory power* of the identifiers or the degree to which record pairs agree. Deterministic approaches typically have high positive predictive value but often suffer from low sensitivity due to the inflexibility of the criteria.

An iterative deterministic approach, such as the well-documented Surveillance, Epidemiology and End Results (SEER)-Medicare algorithm, provides a more flexible alternative to a one-time deterministic approach. It involves an initial match on the most conservative matching criteria, followed by subsequent matches where record pairs that failed to meet the initial criteria are passed to a second, more lenient set of matching criteria. Record pairs that meet the matching criteria at any step are classified as matches, while record pairs that meet no matching criteria are classified as nonmatches. This approach is more flexible and more sensitive than the one-time deterministic approach. In scenarios in which no single unique identifier (e.g., beneficiary ID or SSN) is both available and complete but high-quality direct identifiers are available (e.g., names, dates of birth), the SEER-Medicare algorithm has demonstrated high reliability and validity.

In many cases, identifiers are available but incomplete, fraught with typographical errors, or imperfectly measured. In these scenarios, probabilistic techniques are recommended, as they have consistently outperformed deterministic techniques in earlier research. As described in Chapter 4, a probabilistic approach incorporates the differential discriminatory power of the identifiers and the degree to which two records agree into the agreement and disagreement weights for each identifier. This approach can be used to initially test and validate the discriminatory power of each available identifier. During the linking process, probabilistic methods assign an agreement weight when identifiers agree or a disagreement weight when identifiers disagree, and then derive an overall match score based on the sum of all weights. While probabilistic methods often outperform deterministic methods in information-poor scenarios, they require significantly more time, effort, and technical resources to implement.

An optimal approach that covers all scenarios, datasets, research questions, and/or situations does not exist. Often, as outlined in Chapter 5, combining probabilistic and deterministic methods can be more efficient and save computational resources. For example, a deterministic match on all direct identifiers can be executed first to identify certain matches and the remaining discordant pairs can be evaluated using probabilistic matching. The decision of which approach to use depends ultimately on the research question and the available resources.

Evaluation and Validation of Record Linkage

Irrespective of the linkage method applied, careful evaluation of the output is needed. This begins with a manual review process. Review involves several steps, the first of which involves looking for and resolving ties in which multiple record pairs identified as matches by the algorithm have exactly the same set of values. Next, a random sample of the set of potential matches identified during the blocking phase should be reviewed to evaluate the accuracy of the algorithm and identify circumstances in which the algorithm can be refined to account for complicated cases or unforeseen patterns. Following the manual review process, the final proportion of matches should be compared to known metrics or expected (a priori) estimates. A substantial difference in the observed number of matches versus the expected number of matches is a good indication that the linkage approach needs adjustment.

Recommendations for Reporting Results

Data linkage is a complex process that involves many decisions that may affect the validity and generalizability of the newly linked data source. We recommend that researchers who implement a data linkage to generate an analytic dataset report the results of their data linkage process in manuscripts that utilize the linked data. Specifically, we recommend that researchers use sensitivity, positive predictive value, and the f-measure to characterize the accuracy of the reported strategy. Specificity and negative

Chapter 6. Project Summary and Recommendations for Researchers

predictive value, frequently reported in health services research, will be inflated because of the large number of true nonmatches and thus should not be reported. The metrics should be clearly presented for any algorithm so potential users can weigh their priorities (e.g., sensitivity over positive predictive value) and choose a strategy based on the needs of the specific project. These measures could be reported in the methods sections of manuscripts that utilize the linked data.

Following the matching process, researchers should determine whether there are any important differences in the characteristics of people who are matched and those who are unmatched. The extent to which unmatched individuals differ from matched individuals should be reported in manuscripts using the linked data. This is particularly important when researchers link existing cohorts with external data sources. If the original data source has been used extensively (for example, SEER-Medicare), then identifying any differences between the original (known) cohort and the new cohort is critical to providing transparency to the reader regarding changes in the underlying population post linkage.

Framework for Registry-to-Claims Linkage

We provide several checklists for researchers to use for registry-to-claims linkage project planning and execution. These are conceptualized as (1) project planning, or what you need to consider before applying for funding; and (2) project execution, or what steps you need to take in order to successfully execute the research project.

Project Planning Checklist

[ ] Appropriateness and feasibility

Correct data for research question? Will I have linkage variables, overlap in population? Adequate return on investment (ROI)? Is there enough overlap between datasets? Are additional data elements/variables obtained from completing the linkage of high quality (nonmissing, available on a majority of individuals) on the linked population [effort to link = appropriate gains in data/population]?

[ ] Data ownership and governance

Do the data sources allow for the scope of the proposed work? Are there existing data-governance processes in place? If needed, did the subjects consent to the research?

[ ] Technical environment

Do I have plans to build or leverage a technical environment compliant with security needs? Do I have enough computing power? Do I have enough storage and tools to handle big data?

[ ] Team, skills, and expertise

Do I have access to a team or existing organizational entities for all aspects of the project: data management, information confidentiality and security, linking expertise, epidemiologic expertise (re: selection bias, design, etc.)?

[ ] Cost

Do I have estimates on the cost for advanced expertise? Are the costs for the technical platform feasible over the duration of the project? Do I build or "rent"? Can I leverage aspects of the project to attract followup funding?

Project Execution Checklist

[ ] Build data partnerships and develop Data Use Agreements

Identify stakeholders, including necessary legal, regulatory, or administrative staff. Identify regulatory/security requirements. Develop legal documents/agreements approved by all stakeholders.

[ ] Identify and recruit people with the required technical skills and expertise

Find IT systems partner, data security officer, data manager, linkage programmer, epidemiologic/population expert to help guide decisionmaking.

Linking Data for Health Services Research

[ ] Identify and evaluate available identifiers/linkage keys

Determine the completeness and quality of variables needed for linkage. Evaluate missing, invalid, or unlikely values. Use this assessment to determine the appropriate data linkage strategy.

[ ] Standardize and clean linkage keys

Obtain and review ALL reference documentation available from data partners/vendors or published elsewhere (literature search, gray literature). Outline the standardization protocol for each identifier. Identify any secondary software or datasets (crosswalk files) you need to standardize or clean. Amount of cleaning required will depend on the quality and source of the data.

[ ] Develop a common data model/normalize data

Determine the entity relationships (one to many/one to one), standardize common variables across datasets (e.g., sex, race), standardize formatting (e.g., dates set to mmddyyyy), standardize case (e.g., all uppercase) and punctuation (e.g., remove dashes from SSN), determine how to handle missing values and duplicates.

[ ] Design linkage approach

By incorporating information from the previous steps, decide whether a deterministic linkage strategy is feasible by evaluating any direct identifiers for quality and completeness. Often probabilistic methods or a combined approach must be applied. Evaluate whether and how a "blocking strategy" can be used to improve efficiency and computing requirements. Be sure to incorporate necessary iterative processes, including specific steps for review/evaluation.

[ ] Evaluate/validate record linkage and reporting of linkage metrics

Conduct a manual review of match decisions. The extent and sampling of this review may vary and will be defined by the chosen linkage strategy. Compare results with target or reference populations. Calculate and report statistical measures of performance: sensitivity, positive predictive value, and f-measure.

References

1. Clancy CM, Slutsky JR. Commentary: a progress report on AHRQ's Effective Health Care Program. Health Serv Res. 2007 Oct;42(5):xi-xix. PMID: 17850519.

2. Institute of Medicine. Initial National Priorities for Comparative Effectiveness Research. Washington, DC: National Academies Press; 2009.

3. Congressional Budget Office. Research on the Comparative Effectiveness of Medical Treatments: Issues and Options for an Expanded Federal Role. Pub. No. 2975. Washington, DC; 2007.

4. Smith S. Preface. Med Care. 2007;45 (10 Suppl 2):S1-S2.

5. Sox HC, Greenfield S. Comparative effectiveness research: a report from the Institute of Medicine. Ann Intern Med. 2009;151(3): 203-5. PMID: 19567618.

6. VanLare JM, Conway PH, Sox HC. Five next steps for a new national program for comparative-effectiveness research. N Engl J Med. 2010;362(11): 970-3. PMID: 20164480.

7. Bloomrosen M, Detmer D. Advancing the framework: use of health data--a report of a working conference of the American Medical Informatics Association. J Am Med Inform Assoc. 2008 Nov-Dec;15(6):715-22. PMID: 18755988.

8. Centers for Disease Control and Prevention. FOA: Enhancing Cancer Registry Data for Comparative Effectiveness Research. Atlanta, GA; 2010.

9. Sturmer T, Jonsson Funk M, Poole C, et al. Nonexperimental comparative effectiveness research using linked healthcare databases. Epidemiology. 2011;22(3):298-301. PMID: 21464649.

10. Institute of Medicine. Engineering a Learning Healthcare System: A Look at the Future: Workshop Summary. Washington, DC: National Academies Press; 2011.

11. Blakely T, Salmond C. Probabilistic record linkage and a method to calculate the positive predictive value. Int J Epidemiol. 2002;31(6):1246-52. PMID: 12540730.

12. Bohensky MA, Jolley D, Sundararajan V, et al. Data linkage: a powerful research tool with potential problems. BMC Health Serv Res. 2010;10:346. PMID: 21176171.

13. Howe GR. Use of computerized record linkage in cohort studies. Epidemiol Rev. 1998;20(1):112-21. PMID: 9762514.

14. Lipscomb J, Gotay C, Snyder C. Outcomes Assessment in Cancer: Measures, Methods, and Applications. Cambridge: Cambridge University Press; 2005.

15. Brookhart MA, Sturmer T, Glynn RJ, et al. Confounding control in healthcare database research: challenges and potential approaches. Med Care. 2010;48(6 Suppl):S114-20. PMID: 20473199.

16. Gliklich R, Dreyer N, eds. Registries for Evaluating Patient Outcomes: A User's Guide. AHRQ Publication No. 07-EHC001-1. Agency for Healthcare Research and Quality: Rockville, MD; 2007.

17. Jutte DP, Roos LL, Brownell MD. Administrative record linkage as a tool for public health research. Annu Rev Public Health. 2011;32:91-108. PMID: 21219160.

18. Mortensen PB. The untapped potential of case registers and record-linkage studies in psychiatric epidemiology. Epidemiol Rev. 1995;17(1):205-9. PMID: 8521938.

19. Warren JL, Feuer E, Potosky AL, et al. Use of Medicare hospital and physician data to assess breast cancer incidence. Med Care. 1999;37(5):445-56. PMID: 10335747.

20. Hummler HD, Poets C. [Mortality of extremely low birthweight infants - large differences between quality assurance data and the national birth/death registry]. Z Geburtshilfe Neonatol. 2011;215(1):10-17. PMID: 21344345.

21. Li Q, Glynn RJ, Dreyer NA, et al. Validity of claims-based definitions of left ventricular systolic dysfunction in Medicare patients. Pharmacoepidemiol Drug Saf. 2011;20(7):700-8. PMID: 21608070.

22. Setoguchi S, Solomon DH, Glynn RJ, et al. Agreement of diagnosis and its date for hematologic malignancies and solid tumors between Medicare claims and cancer registry data. Cancer Causes Control. 2007;18(5):561-9. PMID: 17447148.

23. Stürmer T, Schneeweiss S, Avorn J, et al. Adjusting effect estimates for unmeasured confounding with validation data using propensity score calibration. Am J Epidemiol. 2005;162(3):279-89. PMID: 15987725.

24. Winglee M, Valliant R, Schuren F. A case study in record linkage. Survey Methodol. 2005;31(1): 3-11.

25. Pentecost MJ. HIPAA and the law of unintended consequences. J Am Coll Radiol. 2004;1(3):164-5. PMID: 17411551.

26. Dracup K, Bryan-Brown CW. The law of unintended consequences. Am J Crit Care. 2004;13(2):97-9. PMID: 15043236.

27. Kulynych J, Korn D. The new HIPAA (Health Insurance Portability and Accountability Act of 1996) Medical Privacy Rule: help or hindrance for clinical research? Circulation. 2003;108(8):912-4. PMID: 12939240.

28. Salem DN, Pauker SG. The adverse effects of HIPAA on patient care. N Engl J Med. 2003;349(3):309. PMID: 12867622.

29. Kulynych J, Korn D. The new federal medical-privacy rule. N Engl J Med. 2002;347(15):1133-4. PMID: 12374872.

30. Beebe TJ, Ziegenfuss JY, St. Sauver JL, et al. Health Insurance Portability and Accountability Act (HIPAA) authorization and survey nonresponse bias. Med Care. 2011;49(4):365-70. PMID: 21368682.

31. Institute of Medicine. Beyond the HIPAA Privacy Rule: Enhancing Privacy, Improving Health Through Research. Washington, DC: National Academies Press; 2009.

32. Bradley CJ, Penberthy L, Devers KJ, et al. Health services research and data linkages: issues, methods, and directions for the future. Health Serv Res. 2010;45(5 Pt 2):1468-88. PMID: 21054367.

33. Fellegi IP, Sunter AB. A theory for record linkage. J Am Stat Assoc. 1969; 64(328):1183-210.

34. Safran C, Bloomrosen M, Hammond WE, et al. Toward a national framework for the secondary use of health data: an American Medical Informatics Association White Paper. J Am Med Informat Assoc. 2007;14(1):1-9. PMID: 17077452.

35. Hammill BG, Hernandez AF, Peterson ED, et al. Linking inpatient clinical registry data to Medicare claims data using indirect identifiers. Am Heart J. 2009;157(6):995-1000. PMID: 19464409.

36. Tromp M, Ravelli AC, Bonsel GJ, et al. Results from simulated data sets: probabilistic record linkage outperforms deterministic record linkage. J Clin Epidemiol. 2011;64(5):565-72. PMID: 20952162.

37. Keyhani S, Woodward M, Federman AD. Physician views on the use of comparative effectiveness research: a national survey. Ann Intern Med. 2010;153(8):551-2. PMID: 20956718.

38. Sox HC. Comparative effectiveness research: a progress report. Ann Intern Med. 2010;153(7):469-72. PMID: 20679544.

39. Sox HC Helfland M, Grimshaw J, et al. Comparative effectiveness research: challenges for medical journals. J Clin Epidemiol. 2010;63(8):862-4. PMID: 20434882.

40. Newcombe HB, Smith ME, Howe GR, et al. Reliability of computerized versus manual death searches in a study of the health of Eldorado uranium workers. Computers Biol Med. 1983;13(3):157-69. PMID: 6617166.

41. Roos LL, Wajda A. Record linkage strategies. Part 1: estimating information and evaluating approaches. Methods Information Med. 1991;30:117-23. PMID: 1857246.

42. Howe HL, Lake AJ, Shen T. Method to assess identifiability in electronic data files. Am J Epidemiol. 2007;165(5): 597-601. PMID: 17182982.

43. Cook LJ, Olson LM, Dean JM. Probabilistic record linkage: relationships between file sizes, identifiers, and match weights. Methods Information Med. 2001;40:196-203. PMID: 11501632.

44. Marsolo K. Approaches to facilitate institutional review board approval of multicenter research studies. Med Care. 2012;50 Suppl:S77-81. PMID: 22692264.

45. Quantin C, Bouzelat H, Allaert FA, et al. Automatic record hash coding and linkage for epidemiological follow-up data confidentiality. Methods Information Med. 1998;37(3): 271-7. PMID: 9787628.

46. Quantin C, Bouzelat H, Alleart FA, et al. How to ensure data security of an epidemiological follow up: quality assessment of an anonymous record linkage procedure. Int J Med Informat. 1998;49:117-22. PMID: 9723810.

47. Schneier B. Applied Cryptography, Protocols, Algorithms, and Source Code. Chichester: Wiley; 1994.

48. Dhir R, Patel AA, Winters S, et al. A multidisciplinary approach to honest broker services for tissue banks and clinical data: a pragmatic and practical model. Cancer. 2008;113(7):1705-15. PMID: 18683217.

49. Dwork C. Differential privacy: a survey of results. Theory Applications Models Computation Proc. 2008;4978:1-19.

50. Fienberg S. Confidentiality, privacy and disclosure limitation. In: Encyclopedia of Social Measurement. Academic Press; 2005.

51. Kum HC, Ahalt S, et al. Privacy preserving data integration using decoupled data. In: Security and Privacy in Social Network. Springer; 2012.

52. Kum HC, Krishnamurthy A, Pathak D, et al. Secure Decoupled Linkage (SDLink) System for Building a Social Genome. 2013 IEEE International Conference on Big Data (IEEE BigData 2013); 2013.

53. Kum HC, Krishnamurthy A, Machanavajjhala A, et al. Privacy preserving interactive record linkage (PPIRL). J Am Med Informat Assoc. 2014;21(2): 212-20. PMID: 24201028.

54. Hertzman CP, Meagher N, McGrail KM. Privacy by design at Population Data BC: a case study describing the technical, administrative, and physical controls for privacy-sensitive secondary use of personal information for research in the public interest. J Am Med Informat Assoc. 2013;20(1): 25-8. PMID: 22935136.

55. Gladwell M. The Tipping Point: How Little Things Can Make a Big Difference. Boston: Brown and Company; 2000.

56. Hall KL, Feng AX, Moser RP, et al. Moving the science of team science forward - collaboration and creativity. Am J Prev Med. 2008;35(2): S243-249. PMID: 18619406.

57. Stokols D, Hall KL, Taylor BK, et al. The science of team science - overview of the field and introduction to the supplement. Am J Prev Med. 2008;35(2): S77-89. PMID: 18619407.

58. Roos LL, Wajda A, Nicol JP. The art and science of record linkage methods that work with few identifiers. Comput Biol Med. 1986;16(1):45-57. PMID: 394849.

59. Levenshtein V. Binary codes capable of correcting deletions, insertions and reversals. Soviet Physics Doklady. 1966;10:707-10.

60. Jaro MA. Advances in record linkage methodology as applied to matching the 1985 Census of Tampa, Florida. J Am Stat Assoc. 1989;84(406):414-20.

61. Winkler WE. String comparator metrics and enhanced decision rules in the Fellegi-Sunter model of record linkage. American Statistical Association, Proceedings of the Section on Survey Research Methods; 1990.

62. Wajda A, Roos LL. Simplifying record linkage: software and strategy. Comput Biol Med. 1987;17(4):239-48. PMID: 3665453.

63. Randall SM, Ferrante AM, Boyd JH, et al. The effect of data cleaning on record linkage quality. BMC Med Informat Decis Making. 2013; 13:64. PMID: 23739011.

64. Krewski DA, Wang Y, Bartlett S, et al. The effect of record linkage errors on risk estimates in cohort mortality studies. Survey Methodology. 2005;31(1):13-21.

65. Newcombe HB, Kennedy JM. Record linkage: making maximum use of the discriminating power of identifying information. Communications of the ACM. 1962;5(11):563-6.

66. Rogot E, Feinleib M, Ockay KA, et al. On the feasibility of linking census samples to the National Death Index for epidemiologic studies: a progress report. Am J Public Health. 1983 Nov;73(11):1265-9. PMID: 6625029.

67. Rogot E, Sorlie P, Johnson NJ. Probabilistic methods in matching census samples to the National Death Index. J Chron Dis. 1986;39(9):719-34. PMID: 3734026.

68. Clark DE. Development of a statewide trauma registry using multiple linked sources of data. Proc Annu Symp Comput Appl Med Care. 1993;654-8. PMID: 8130556.

69. Bell RM, Keesey J, Richards T. The urge to merge: linking vital statistics records and Medicaid claims. Med Care.1994 Oct;32(10):1004-18. PMID: 7934268.

70. Clark DE, Hahn DR. Comparison of probabilistic and deterministic record linkage in the development of a statewide trauma registry. Proc Annu Symp Comput Appl Med Care. 1995:397-401. PMID: 8563310.

71. Jamieson E, Roberts J, Browne G. The feasibility and accuracy of anonymized record linkage to estimate shared clientele among three health and social service agencies. Methods Information Med. 1995;34:371-7. PMID: 7476469.

72. Muse AG, Mikl J, Smith PF. Evaluating the quality of anonymous record linkage using deterministic procedures with the New York State AIDS registry and a hospital discharge file. Stat Med. 1995 Mar 15-Apr 15;14(5-7):499-509. PMID: 7792444.

73. Doebbeling BN, Wyant DK, McCoy KD, et al. Linked insurance-tumor registry database for health services research. Med Care. 1999 Nov;37(11):1105-15. PMID: 10549613.

74. Grannis SJ, Overhage JM, Hui S, et al. Analysis of a probabilistic record linkage technique without human review. AMIA 2003 Symposium Proc. 2003:259-63. PMID: 14728174.

75. Weiner M, Stump TE, Callahan CM, et al. A practical method of linking data from Medicare claims and a comprehensive electronic medical records system. Int J Med Informat. 2003;71:57-69. PMID: 12909159.

76. Bradley CJ, Given CW, Luo Z, et al. Medicaid, Medicare, and the Michigan Tumor Registry: a linkage strategy. Med Decis Making. 2007 Jul-Aug;27(4):352-63. PMID: 17641138.

77. Jacobs JP, Edwards FH, Shahian DM, et al. Successful linking of the Society of Thoracic Surgeons adult cardiac surgery database to Centers for Medicare and Medicaid Services Medicare data. Ann Thoracic Surg. 2010;90:1150-7. PMID: 20868806.

78. Nadpara PA, Madhavan SS. Linking Medicare, Medicaid, and cancer registry data to study the burden of cancers in West Virginia. Medicare Medicaid Res Rev. 2012;2(4). PMID: 24800152.

79. Li B, Quan H, Fong A, et al. Assessing record linkage between health care and vital statistics databases using deterministic methods. BMC Health Serv Res. 2006;6(1):1-10. PMID: 16597337.

80. Potosky AL, Riley GF, Lubitz JD, et al. Potential for cancer related health services research using a linked Medicare-tumor registry database. Med Care. 1993;31(8):732-48. PMID: 8336512.

81. Warren JL, Klabunde CN, Schrag D, et al. Overview of the SEER-Medicare data: content, research applications, and generalizability to the

United States elderly population. Med Care. 2002 Aug;40(8 Suppl):IV-3-18. PMID: 12187163.

82. National Cancer Institute SEER-Medicare Program. Search SEER-Medicare Publications. 2011. http://healthservices.cancer.gov/seermedicare/overview/publications.html. Accessed March 4, 2011.

83. Warren J, Carpenter WR (Report Author). Email: Details on SEER-Medicare linkage methods. August 20, 2010.

84. Quantin C, Bouzelat H, Allaert FAA, et al. How to ensure data security of an epidemiological follow up: quality assessment of an anonymous record linkage procedure. Int J Med Informat. 1998;49:117-22. PMID: 9723810.

85. Quantin C, Allaert FA, Avillach P, et al. Building application-related patient identifiers: what solution for a European country? Int J Telemed Applications. 2008:1-5. PMID: 18401447.

86. Christen P, Goiser K. Quality and complexity measures for data linkage and deduplication. Stud Computational Intelligence. 2007;43:127-51.

87. Hernandez MA, Stolfo SJ. The merge/purge for large databases. Proceedings of the SIGMOD 95 Conference; 1995:127-38.

88. Belin TR, Rubin DB. A method for calibrating false matches in record linkage. J Am Stat Assoc. 1995;90:694-707.

89. Dey D, Sarkar S, De P. Entity matching in heterogenous databases: a distance based decision model. Proceedings of the 31st Hawaii International Conference on System Sciences; 1998.

90. Cochinwala M, Kurien V, Lalk G, et al. Efficient Data Reconciliation. Bellcore; 1998.

91. Verykios VS, Moustakides GV. A cost optimal decision model for record matching. Workshop on Data Quality: Challenges for Computer Science and Statistics; 2001.

92. Van Rijsbergen CJ. Information Retrieval: Data Structures and Algorithms. London: Butterworths; 1979.

Abbreviations

AHRQ	Agency for Healthcare Research and Quality	PII	Personally Identifiable Information
		PIN	Personal Identification Number
CER	Comparative effectiveness research	PPIRL	Privacy Preserving Interactive Record Linkage
CPU	Central processing unit		
DUA	Data Use Agreement	PPV	Positive predictive value
DEcIDE	Developing Evidence to Inform Decisions about Effectiveness	RAID	Redundant Array of Independent Disks
DOB	Date of birth	RAM	Random access memory
ePHI	Electronic Protected Health Information	RCT	Randomized controlled trial
		ROI	Return on investment
EM	Expectation-maximization	RPM	Revolutions per minute
FIPS	Federal Information Processing Standards	SAN	Storage Area Network
		SATA	Serial Advance Technology Attachment
FISMA	Federal Information Security Management Act	Serial SCSI or SAS	Serial Attached Small Computer System Interface
GUID	Globally unique identifier		
HIPAA	Health Insurance Portability and Accountability Act	SEER	Surveillance, Epidemiology and End Results
IP	Internet Protocol	SFTP	Secure file transfer protocol
IRB	Institutional Review Board	SHA-2	Secure Hash Algorithm version 2
IT	Information technology	SSD	Solid state disk
LDS	Limited Dataset	SSH	Secure command line
NCCCR	North Carolina Central Cancer Registry	SSN	Social Security Number
		SWOT	Strengths/weaknesses/opportunities/threats
NIST	National Institute for Standards and Technology		
		URL	Universal Resource Locator
NPV	Negative predictive value	USB	Universal Serial Bus
PAYER	Claims data for beneficiaries in privately insured health plans in North Carolina		
PHI	Protected Health Information		

www.ingramcontent.com/pod-product-compliance
Lightning Source LLC
Chambersburg PA
CBHW081734170526
45167CB00009B/3815